Ten Minute Tone-U[p] For Dummies®

D1298896

T

Tone-up/cardio workout

Use this chart if you do your tone-ups 3 days each week. On alternate days include at least 20 minutes of cardio (see Chapter 20). Simply make a copy for each week you work out. You only need four copies to reach your 30-day target date! But you can always make more to reach your long-term goals. Just fill in the blanks with each tone-up exercise you plan to perform each day (see Chapters 17 and 18 for workout menus); begin each day's workout with an aerobic warm-up; record your sets and reps; and on alternate days write in the type and the length of your cardio workouts. Remember to end each workout with a stretch and eat a sensible diet (see Chapter 19).

Week of _____

Day 1 – Tone-Up Workout	Reps	Sets	Day 2 – Cardio Workout	Total minutes
Day 3 – Tone-Up Workout	**Reps**	**Sets**	**Day 4 – Cardio Workout**	**Total minutes**
Day 5 – Tone-Up Workout	**Reps**	**Sets**	**Day 6 – Cardio Workout**	**Total minutes**

Day 7 – Cardio Workout	Total minutes	Notes:

Ten Minute Tone-Ups For Dummies®

Cheat Sheet

Week-long tone-up workout

Use this handy chart for doing your 7-day tone-ups. You only need four photocopies to reach your 30-day target date! But you can always make more to reach your long-term goals. Just fill in the blanks for each tone-up exercise you plan to perform each day (see Chapters 17 and 18 for workout menus). Then begin each day's workout with an aerobic warm-up; record your reps and sets as you do each tone-ups move; and end each day's workout with stretching. Remember to incorporate at least 10 minutes of cardio (see Chapter 20), in addition to your warm-up, at least 3 days a week and eat a sensible diet (see Chapter 19).

Week of _____

Day 1	Reps	Sets	Day 2	Reps	Sets
Day 3	Reps	Sets	Day 4	Reps	Sets
Day 5	Reps	Sets	Day 6	Reps	Sets
Day 7	Reps	Sets	Notes:		

Wiley, the Wiley Publishing logo, For Dummies, the Dummies Man logo, the For Dummies Bestselling Book Series logo and all related trade dress are trademarks or registered trademarks of John Wiley & Sons, Inc. and/or its affiliates. All other trademarks are property of their respective owners.

For Dummies: Bestselling Book Series for Beginners

Ten Minute Tone-Ups

FOR DUMMIES®

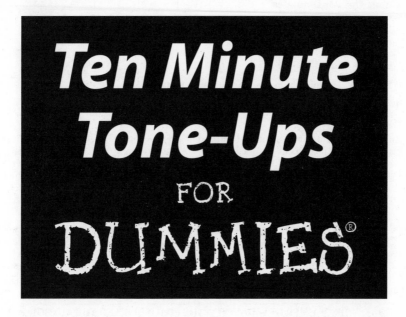

Ten Minute Tone-Ups

FOR DUMMIES®

by Cyndi Targosz

WILEY

Wiley Publishing, Inc.

Ten Minute Tone-Ups For Dummies®

Published by
Wiley Publishing, Inc.
111 River St.
Hoboken, NJ 07030-5774
www.wiley.com

WILEY

About the Author

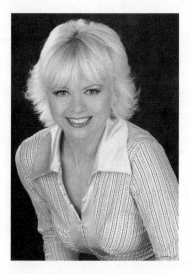

Cyndi Targosz is a nationally recognized lifestyle/fitness expert and motivational speaker. She is certified by ACE, AFAA, and AALC. Her fitness video and audio programs have sold over a half million copies. A graduate of Wayne State University, Cyndi obtained her degree in Speech Pathology and Anatomy and Physiology.

Her background includes work as an actress, model, dancer, radio personality, voiceover artist, and singer. All of these experiences have factored into the elements of Cyndi's core belief of enjoying and having passion in the journey while setting realistic goals. She has successfully exhibited this philosophy into her M.B.S. System (Mind, Body, Spirit) where the mind must be centered, the body must be cared for, and the spirit must be fed. As president and CEO of her own company, STARGLOW Productions Inc., Cyndi's clients have included Hollywood actors, actresses, models, athletes, and other celebrities. Her corporate wellness clientele have included such major firms as Pacific Bell, Kaiser Permanente, Royal Caribbean Cruises, Volkswagen of America, and many others. Contribution of her time and talents have been felt by numerous charitable organizations among them the American Cancer Society, the YWCA, and the Girl Scouts of America. She is a frequent guest expert on numerous radio and television shows. Cyndi's personal philosophy maintains a focus on the interrelationship of balance on the inner and outer glow that provides all-encompassing health, beauty, and wellness. Visit www.starglow.com for more information about Cyndi Targosz.

Dedication

This book is dedicated to my parents Helen and Stanley J. Targosz Sr. who taught me to live life to the fullest!

Author's Acknowledgments

There have been so many wonderful people who have supported me throughout my life and on this project. I wish to extend my sincere gratitude and thanks to all of them.

Thanks to all the talented people from Wiley Publishing who collaborated to bring this book to fruition including: Joyce Pepple, Tracy Bogier, Holly Gastineau-Grimes, Carmen Kirkorian, Michelle Hacker, and Kristin Cocks. Thanks to Mary Bednarek, for her enthusiastic support, my project editor Jennifer Connolly for her guidance, and to Corbin Collins for his positive inspiration and for being the best Dummies mentor ever.

I'd also like to thank my personal assistants Erik Feuchuk, who also was technical director on the photo shoot, and Dimitri Pieries for their long hours and dedication. Thanks to Tobin Bennett for doing a great job on the photography, model Derrick Cox, and my make-up artist Nicole Allen.

To my beautiful family including my parents, two brothers, five sisters, and their spouses, my nieces and nephews, aunts, uncles, and cousins. I love you all.

To my dear friends and associates who have always believed in me and what I stand for: Dr. Jeffrey Anshel, Lila Baron, Alan Benfield-Bush, Marty Bernstein, Debra and David Budge, William Felber, Mike Fisher, Cynthia and Ron Foy, Trudi and Mauri Friedman, Jim Gates, Teri Gianeti-Sergeant, Bill Gladstone, Shirley Goodman, Michael Goodman, Demetria Katsihitis, Paul Kirby, Mark Levin, Bernie and Estelle Meadows, Leslie McClure, Linda and Paul Ottosi, Gary Owens, Mark and Lyn Proffer, Sandy Pollock, Augustus Raney, Gary Ross, Jim Spencer, Kitty Spencer, Sr Seraphine, Anastasia Taylor, Gina Traficant, Elaine Traskos, Sonya VanSickle, Matt Wagner, Beth Young, and all the others too numerous to name who have contributed so much to me along the way.

Publisher's Acknowledgments

We're proud of this book; please send us your comments through our Dummies online registration form located at www.dummies.com/register/.

Some of the people who helped bring this book to market include the following:

Acquisitions, Editorial, and Media Development

Project Editor: Jennifer Connolly

Acquisitions Editor: Tracy Boggier

Copy Editor: Jennifer Connolly

Assistant Editor: Holly Gastineau-Grimes

Technical Editor: Damon Faust

Editorial Manager: Michelle Hacker, Carmen Krikorian

Editorial Assistant: Courtney Allen

Cover Photo: Tobin Bennett

Cartoons: Rich Tennant (www.the5thwave.com)

Composition

Project Coordinator: Maridee Ennis

Layout and Graphics: Brian Drumm, Jacque Roth, Heather Ryan, Brent Savage, Julie Trippetti

Proofreaders: John Greenough, Joseph Niesen, Brian H. Walls, TECHBOOKS Production Services

Indexer: TECHBOOKS Production Services

Publishing and Editorial for Consumer Dummies

Diane Graves Steele, Vice President and Publisher, Consumer Dummies

Joyce Pepple, Acquisitions Director, Consumer Dummies

Kristin A. Cocks, Product Development Director, Consumer Dummies

Michael Spring, Vice President and Publisher, Travel

Brice Gosnell, Associate Publisher, Travel

Kelly Regan, Editorial Director, Travel

Publishing for Technology Dummies

Andy Cummings, Vice President and Publisher, Dummies Technology/General User

Composition Services

Gerry Fahey, Vice President of Production Services

Debbie Stailey, Director of Composition Services

Contents at a Glance

Table of Contents

Introduction

- -

*F*ast food! Fast cars! Fast computers! And yes . . . fast fitness! In the time it takes you to wolf down a pint of ice cream, you can work at trimming your thighs, shaping your chest, toning your tummy — and still have time for a healthy portion of a "little dessert." Is this some crazy quick-fix scheme? Hardly. *Ten Minute Tone-Ups For Dummies* is a safe and sensible program that promises to help you look and feel better in 30 days. It consists of doing the workout daily and following sound nutritional advice.

I have to point out right away that you cannot spot reduce. Fat doesn't just melt away in one particular body area. However, experts agree that you can tone up underlying muscles and therefore target trouble spots. This book makes it possible to get quick results, but you also get many added benefits: new energy, a better attitude about yourself, help in making healthy food choices, and more.

I start with the question: Why did you pick up this book? Did it finally happen? The invitation! Not just any invitation, but *the invitation.* You know, the class reunion, the wedding, the let's-take-a-cruise invitation. The one that makes grown men cry and women squeeeeeze into jeans that are so tight they are convinced the cleaners shrank them. Perhaps you are desperately trying to turn back the hands of time, or maybe you really do love and care about yourself. Whatever your reason for starting this program, Good for you, and I hope you use it as a kick-start to get and stay motivated.

In this book, I help you get ready for a new, active lifestyle, show you how to set realistic goals, and prepare you to take action. I explain the different body types and talk about muscle fiber makeup using simple descriptions. That way, you can be clear as to what you can and cannot expect when targeting trouble spots as you go through this program.

The meat of this book is the ten minute tone-ups themselves. You can choose between several fun, fast, and full-course fitness menus that target one trouble spot, or several muscles, or your whole body. There's a lot of variety to keep you from getting bored.

If there's any panic within you as you embark on this 30-day toning time, lay it to rest. This book is chock full of information that can give you the confidence to reach your target date with flying colors. Of course, even better is to take it beyond 30 days into a lifetime of total wellness. Good luck!

How to Use This Book

Ten Minute Tone-Ups For Dummies is a very user-friendly book. You do not have to read it from left to right or from the beginning to the end, though you can if you so desire. You can start at the beginning, the middle, or the final pages. It's up to you. Hopefully, the book won't wind up as a beer coaster.

This book is modular. Think of each page as a window of opportunity. Loaded with tips and information, on most pages you see cross references that point to other windows of opportunity (other pages, in this case). This format is meant to be interactive, meaning that *you* play a major role in customizing your workout to meet *your* personal needs. Following are some suggestions on how you can use the book to reach your goals:

 ✔ **Getting an overview:** If you are new to exercise, I suggest you read Parts I and VI first. Part I can help you get an overview of the world of working out before you start so that you are familiar with terms and equipment needed. I show you how to set realistic goals and how to prepare so that you can have a safe, successful workout. Part VI is loaded with motivation and fitness-scheduling tips. You can then hit the tone-ups in the other parts.

 ✔ **Using the body parts part:** If you have exercised before, you may choose to target one or more particular body parts. Part II of this book focuses on the upper body, Part III on the lower body, and Part IV on your core (abs and lower back). Be aware that if you were to do all of the exercises included for one particular body part, your tone-up would go over 10 minutes. Therefore, select four or five moves if you need to stay in that timesaving framework.

 ✔ **Customizing:** Whether you are new to exercise or advanced, Part V can help you create a program that is 10 minutes, 20 minutes, or more. Choose from several fitness menus that you can mix together in different ways for variety. It also discusses healthy food choices as well as the importance of a cardio workout.

How This Book Is Organized

Ten Minute Tone-Ups For Dummies is organized to save you time. Feel free to open any page, chapter, or part in whatever order you desire. Following is a brief description about each of the six parts to help you decide which section you want to hit first.

Part 1: Get Ready, Get Set, Get Active!

This part is the nuts and bolts of the program. It provides an overview of the many ways you can tone up. Whether you choose to stick with a 10-minute plan or venture out to a longer workout, this part helps you to get the most out of this plan for improving your life. I remind you to respect your medical limitations and help you set goals. You'll have fun discovering what your body type is and how you can emphasize your strong points and downplay the lesser-liked areas. There's a whole chapter dedicated to stretching. Use it in conjunction with all your tone-ups, or follow it on its own to relax, rejuvenate, and increase flexibility. The philosophy of mind-body fitness and the power of positive visualization are introduced in this part. These concepts may sound New-Agey, but they really can boost your results significantly. Finally, I give you an opportunity to make a sincere commitment to truly tone up in 30 days by providing a handy ten minute tone-ups commitment contract that you can sign and send to me. Doing so can help to keep you focused on and committed to your goals.

Part 11: Upper-Body Workouts

If your goal is to work on your chest, upper back, shoulders, or arms, this part is for you. For each area of focus, I provide a brief explanation of what the corresponding muscles are called and what they do. The muscle illustrations help you visualize what is going on as you work your muscles, which can enhance the effectiveness of your tone-ups.

Toning up doesn't have to be boring: I offer numerous exercises for plenty of variety. I chose movements that, when taken together, can sculpt your entire upper body. Take advantage of the tips sprinkled here and there to help you with breathing and posture. And I give several options for each exercise to enhance or intensify your workout by letting you adjust to your skill level.

Part 111: Lower-Body Workouts

This part gets to the bottom of body part problem areas. It includes an intensive array of exercises that target your thighs, hamstrings, quads, buns, and calves. This part includes several moves that can be done anywhere to help you save time and speed up results. Each exercise comes with tips to help you execute the moves in optimum form. Peruse the other options for variety. There are also suggestions that modify the moves to different levels of difficulty. If an exercise is too hard to execute, for example, you can take advantage of the options provided to still get something out of it. Likewise, if the exercise becomes too easy, I offer lots of ways to keep you challenged. As you progress, you can move on to more advanced movements.

Part IV: Core: Abs and Lower Back

Perfect abs are no doubt on everyone's wish list. Part IV can show you how to achieve your personal best obliques as well as defined upper and lower abs (which are actually one long muscle). Here you also find plenty of safe lower-back exercises. It is the combination of abs and lower-back moves that make up your *core.* A strong core provides the stability to not only make your abs the best they can be but the rest of your body as well. There are several tips on breathing that can help you make exercises such as The Crunch gets results faster than if you didn't breathe properly. Utilize the other options I include to custom-make your workout. That way you can have some variety or match your level of skill.

Part V: Customizing Your Workout and Maximizing Your Results

Workouts don't work if you can't integrate them into your lifestyle. Ten minute tone-ups are totally interactive, and this part offers plenty of suggestions to help you customize your plan. Nowadays, it seems like much of our lives are out of our control — but not this program. In this part, you are in the driver's seat. I provide lots of ten minute fast-fitness "menus" that you can use just as they are — or mix them up for variety. I give you a good selection of full-course fitness menus so that, if inspired, you can expand your workout to 20 minutes or longer. Not to be left out is the chapter dedicated to nutrition. Following this nourishing advice can speed up your tone-up goals. To maximize your results even more, there is a chapter that explains the benefits of cardiovascular fitness and offers several aerobic choices. If your lifestyle takes you out of town, the chapter on traveling fit and well has plenty of tips to take on the road.

Part VI: The Part of Tens

This part is a potpourri of topics that can add to your workout. For example: motivational pitfalls. Perhaps you are dealing with body-image or low self-esteem problems, lack of willpower, or lack of time. I offer suggestions here to help you overcome these obstacles. If your schedule is so tight that even ten minutes doesn't seem doable, check out my scheduling tips. And, because you may as well look your best as you tone up, I give you my top ten favorite workout-wear manufacturers, including loads of information on quality products that are functional as well as stylish.

Conventions Used in This Book

Following are conventions that are used throughout the book. They are consistent and easy to follow.

- ✔ If a word appears in *italics* you can expect a description that is not too complicated.
- ✔ Web addresses can be found in `this font`.
- ✔ Cross references are often in parenthesis (like this), or are simply given in the text.
- ✔ Sidebars, in shaded boxes throughout the book, are not integral to the chapter that they subside in, but provide lots of useful or interesting ancillary information.

Icons in This Book

These catchy little drawings can grab your attention when there is no time to waste.

This is my favorite icon — when you see it, you know that there is an exercise that can be done anywhere and just about anytime, such as at work during a break or while sitting at your computer.

This icon gives you the heads up on how to breathe. Proper breathing helps your body work efficiently during an exercise. To remember the technique I give breathing a XXX rating: eXhale on eXertion during eXercise.

Proper form ensures safety and good results, whereas poor, slouching, or sloppy posture can derail your goals quickly — or worse, cause injury. The posture patrol icon alerts you to the aligned position your body needs to be in.

Tips are always-helpful tidbits of advice that help you execute an exercise better or provide additional important information to a topic being covered.

The warning icon beckons you to proceed with caution. For example, if a move done wrong would be dangerous, the warning icon signals how to avoid that.

 The Technical Stuff icon flags jargon that can make you sound like a pro if you use it. Words like *rectus abdominis* or *gluteus maximus* may scare you now, but they always have simple explanations and can make you impressive at your next social engagement.

 When an important tidbit might be easily forgotten, the Remember icon jolts your memory.

Where to Go from Here

I invite you to dive into this book. Have fun searching these pages in any order you like. No rules! Enjoy every moment, every minute, every ten minute tone-up.

Part I
Get Ready, Get Set, Get Active!

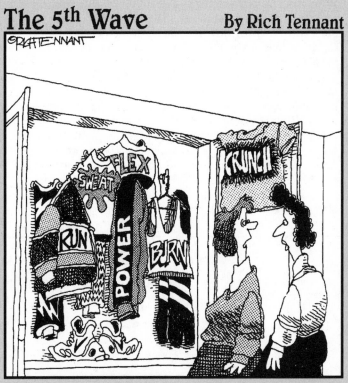

The 5th Wave   By Rich Tennant

"I'm not sure I can live up to my workout clothes."

In this part . . .

*J*ust by picking up this book, you have already begun to make a positive change — good for you! My program really works, but you have to make the commitment and stick with it. I provide a Ten Minute Tone-Ups Commitment Contract that, if you choose, you can sign and send to me. In this part, I also give you the tools to stick with the program by showing you how to prepare for the work you must do and by explaining how to overcome setbacks. I also guide you toward loving your natural self and then explain how to set realistic personal goals based on your body type. I even give you advice on equipment, terminology, what to wear, where to exercise, and even choosing music. My secret is to take you where you are now and get you to an overall healthier lifestyle. If you're not pumped yet, you can find some great ways in this part to get and stay motivated — so let's get started!

Chapter 1

Maximizing Ten Minutes for Life

. . . .

In This Chapter

▶ Looking at the whole picture

▶ Zeroing in on specific trouble spots

▶ Considering medical and safety matters

▶ Choosing an active healthy lifestyle

▶ Benefiting from mind-body focus

. . . .

Are you ready? Ready to get set, make goals, and devise a plan of action? What is it that you personally want to achieve in the next 30 days and beyond? Taking ten minutes a day for yourself can be the most productive time you ever spend. In this chapter, I share some top timesaving tips. I also help you target your trouble spots — don't worry, everybody's got them. And I address health and safety issues; it's important to respect your medical limitations. Discover the rejuvenating benefits of connecting your mind and body — a motivating factor to be jazzed about. Making activity and a healthy diet a part of your everyday life can be very rewarding. Take it to the max.

Getting an Overview of the Basics

Deciding to make a positive lifestyle change is a very important first step. Here is a basic overview of what's needed to meet your ten minute tone-up health and fitness goals.

Creating your ten minute interactive workout

Ten minute tone-ups is an exciting, fun, personal, and user-friendly program. You can create it however you like, so it works for your individual needs and schedule (see Chapter 2 for more on scheduling ten minute 30-day workouts).

Whether you choose to work on one body part or several, it's all at your fingertips. You can flip to a specific chapter that targets what you want to work on, or use moves from several chapters mixed up.

Doing an entire body part chapter can take much longer than ten minutes, so pace yourself accordingly. Select four or five moves to stay within the ten minute time framework, though of course if you have more time, go for it.

Another interactive option is to take advantage of the prepackaged fast-fitness menus I include in Chapter 17. Have fun mixing them up for variety. From these menus, order the body part that works for you. Include stretching and cardio moves to totally speed up your results (see Chapters 4 and 20 for more on these important workout elements).

Creating a 20-minute or longer plan

I'm so convinced that you can succeed at and will enjoy doing your ten minute tone-ups, I invite you to challenge yourself even more. Why not create a 20-minute or more plan? The health benefits of longer workouts are enormous, plus they really speed up your results. If you are going to use the old "I don't have time" excuse, try this tip: Keep doing your ten minute tone-ups daily, but pick out a day or two in which you attempt a more extensive workout. Gradually increase how often you do a 20-minute or more plan, and your body will adapt. Don't stress about how to do this — check out the prepackaged full-course fitness menus in Chapter 18. Another option is to do more than one ten minute tone-up session in a day. Studies show that doing short sessions more than once a day can be substantially beneficial.

I have a client who recently lost 50 pounds in one year. He expressed to me that since he discovered how good he feels being in shape by doing longer exercise increments, he's never wanted to go back to his old habits. On days when he lacks motivation, his desire to look and feel great wins out.

Giving it your best stretch

Some people never stretch, other than at the seventh inning of a baseball game. Reaching for peanuts and Crackerjacks requires some flexibility, but hardly enough to satisfy your stretching needs. If you strike out stretching from your ten minute tone-ups routine, you lose. Stretching helps your body work more efficiently and speeds up results right off the bat. Stretching also increases your flexibility and helps to keep you injury free — a winning combo. Then there are the rejuvenating effects. For an entire array of stretches, slide into Chapter 4.

Including a cardio workout

To totally maximize your **ten minute tone-ups,** of course, you'll want to include a cardiovascular workout, which means aerobic exercise. A cardio workout can speed up fat loss while helping your muscles to work more efficiently as you tone up. Jog over to Chapter 20 for the scoop on aerobic exercise, selecting a cardio workout, and the importance of finding your target heart rate and monitoring your pulse.

Always include a cardio or aerobic warm-up before your ten minute tone-ups to get the circulation going and help avoid injury.

Targeting Your Trouble Spots

I am always a trumpeter for overall general health and fitness. However, with a 30-day target date, it's certainly okay to hone in on specific trouble spots. Heck, everybody has one or more problem areas. Decide what part or parts you want to tone up? Your legs, thighs? Just don't say wings.

Replacing fat with firm muscles

Unfortunately, you cannot spot reduce. For example, doing hundreds of crunches simply will not make your stomach magically disappear. Sorry! When you lose weight, it comes off your entire body. This does not mean you should dis crunches. Sit up and take notice: Doing crunches, like doing any of the ten minute tone-ups in this book, firms and tones underlying muscles while burning overall body fat. That's good news. To replace fat with firm muscles, do the following.

✔ **Burn fat:** Including an aerobic activity in your routine burns fat and accelerates your toned-up results (see Chapter 20 for adding a cardio workout).

✔ **Do your ten minute tone-ups:** Be sure to do your personalized tone-ups (see Chapters 17 and 18 for a fun selection of fast- and full-course fitness menus).

✔ **Eat a balanced diet:** Escalate your results with a balanced diet (check out Chapter 19).

Are ten minutes enough?

Are ten minutes of exercising enough to get any benefit? In a word — yes! In fact, many experts believe that if done properly, a short workout achieves better results than a longer workout done poorly. For each of the exercises in this book, I carefully explain how to get ready, how to do the move, and how to explore other options so you are sure to meet your level of difficulty. Each exercise is illustrated with photos. With a 30-day target date, though, it is critical that you stick to your plan if you expect results.

Using good technique makes a ten minute tone-up better than a sloppy half-hour workout. However, squeezing in 20 minutes or more of exercise with good technique is extremely beneficial. When done correctly you can burn more calories and speed up the rate at which results are noticed.

Addressing Medical, Health, and Safety Issues

When starting a fitness program, it's important to take stock of your general wellness. Addressing medical, health, and safety concerns ensures that you end up doing the appropriate program at the level of difficulty that is best for you. The following is established wisdom.

Checking in with your doctor

It's always a good idea to see your physician before starting any exercise program, and getting one before starting your ten minute tone-ups makes sense for your safety and general health. Besides, getting an annual physical should be part of your preventive medicine plan. The doctor can determine if you are at risk for cardiovascular disease, musculoskeletal problems, or if you have other health issues. He or she can sort through possible symptoms of heart problems, orthopedic aches, pregnancy, and so forth. All of this information helps you to take responsibility of your own body so that you can accommodate any medical limitations.

When consulting with your physician, take along a copy of your ten minute tone-ups plan. She can use it to advise you of what is appropriate or not for you, should you have any limitations. Your doctor will probably offer encouragement to you on your fitness journey.

Knowing your medical limitations

For safety reasons, always be aware of your medical limitations. It's important to respect any current injuries or health problems. For example, let's say your goal is to sculpt your shoulders and arms for an upcoming pool party. Under normal circumstances that would be a reasonable goal. However, if you recently injured your shoulder swinging a bat at a weekend warrior baseball game, this could be cause for medical concern. Trying to sculpt your arms after such an injury may not be appropriate because shoulder movement would be involved. You'd be better off seeing a physician. Depending on the extent of the injury, you might be able to adapt your goals to include a cardio workout and lower-body and core tone-ups rather than arm and shoulder exercises. Respect any injury or medical problem you have. Nobody knows your body like you do.

Preventing back problems

Primary care physicians see people with back problems back to back. Lower-back problems are the second-leading cause for doctor's office visits after colds. Approximately 80 percent of adults end up with lower-back pain. That figure is astounding when you consider that many of those problems can be prevented.

Most back problems are caused by weak muscles surrounding the spine. With weak postural muscles, any chance for correct body mechanics goes kaput. And it certainly doesn't help if you slouch all the time. Did you just sit up or stand up straight when I said that? Good. Following are some great suggestions to prevent back problems:

- ✔ **Strengthening your core:** Strengthening your core muscles (lower back and abs) creates stability for your back and entire body. (I've packed Part IV of this book with core moves.)

- ✔ **Do resistance training:** Doing weight training, such as that provided in ten minute tone-ups, helps maintain bone density.

- ✔ **Maintain appropriate weight:** It's common for overweight people to develop back problems. Try to maintain an appropriate weight. See Chapter 2 for testing body-fat composition and how to create goals after fitness testing.

- ✔ **Do stretching moves:** Stretching can help prevent back problems. Muscles to stretch include hamstrings, hip flexors, back, abs, and chest. Bet you didn't realize so many muscles affected your back! (See Chapter 4 for several back-saving stretches.)

Posture pointers

Proper posture can make all the difference in the world to your total look and health. Unfortunately, it's way too easy to cave into that very unflattering position I call "poor posture slump." You know — the one that occurs when you sit in front of the TV, drive, or even stand. The shoulders droop, and your spine collapses into a rounded bend. Poor posture can also ruin the results of your ten minute tone-ups by working the wrong muscles or, worse yet, causing injury. It's time to straighten up!

Posture is how all your body parts work together, whether you are sitting, standing, exercising, or doing anything else. To achieve good posture, your feet should be planted on the floor parallel to each other. Put your chest out and bring your shoulders slightly back but relaxed. Hold your abs in tight and keep your butt tucked under. Here are some helpful posture pointers:

- ✔ **Elongate the spine:** Pretend you are a marionette and a tight rope is pulling at you from above and below.

- ✔ **Keep your chin parallel to the floor:** This can help make the look of a double chin disappear.

- ✔ **Distribute your weight evenly:** Pointing your toes forward rather than outward helps maintain stability.

- ✔ **Hold your head up:** Holding your head up as if to lengthen your neck can make your neck appear longer, and you look taller.

Making Activity and a Healthy Diet Part of Everyday Life

Life is so much more enjoyable when you feel your best. Being active and eating right can bridge the gap between merely existing and really living. Use this opportunity to take your ten minute tone-ups to the max. Forget fitness and diet fads — choose to be active and eat healthy.

Forgetting fitness myths

There are so many myths out there that should be squashed. I'll list a few. Stamp them out immediately.

- ✔ **Spot-reduction myth:** You *cannot* spot reduce no matter what the false ads say. You *can* tone up and lose overall body fat (see "Targeting Your Trouble Spots" earlier in this chapter).

- ✔ **Light weights bulking myth:** Somehow over the years people, especially women, became afraid of lifting light weights for fear of bulking up too much. This is false. Unless you take steroids and do extensive power lifting, you cannot bulk up like that. Most people do not have the genetics for such extreme pump-up action (see Chapter 2 for more on muscle fiber makeup). If you are doing only one or two sets with light weights, you should not notice a huge increase in muscle size, yet you can tone up, burn calories and build stronger bones and muscles.

- ✔ **Exercise weakens the heart myth:** This one really amazes me. Exercise does not weaken the heart. It can help to make it stronger.

- ✔ **Toning up does not help you reduce weight myth:** Toning up actually helps to increase your metabolism. And a faster metabolism means faster weight loss.

Forgetting fad diets

Fad diets are so prevalent in our culture that it can be difficult to differentiate between what is sound information and what isn't. In fact, fad diet pseudo facts are reported on the news as if they were the gospel truth. It's okay to be aware of new diet information, but choose a healthy diet based on facts that are proven to be good for you. For example, eating only cabbage may help you lose weight, but you shortchange yourself of many necessary nutrients. See "Choosing a healthy diet" later in this chapter and Chapter 19.

Boosting your current activity level

Boosting your current activity level can certainly speed up your tone-up results, but it also has long-term benefits that warrant your attention. In 1996, the Surgeon General's report proclaimed that regular physical activity performed on most days of the week reduces the risk of developing or dying from some of the leading causes of illness and death in the United States. What does that mean to you? You can have fun, be active, and stay healthy at the same time. Here's how:

- ✔ **Create a daily activity log:** Start keeping track of all physical activities when you do them. Jot them down in a notebook, computer, or whatever works for you. Include everything from washing the car to playing with the kids.

- ✔ **Select new and fun activities:** Think of ways you can incorporate new activities into your life. Be creative! For example, I come from a big family with lots of brother and sisters. We often do group fun stuff such as laser tag, miniature golf, and even bowling. We laugh, have fun, and are active.

✔ **Evaluate your log:** Once a week review your log. See if you find any patterns, such as sluggish Mondays or no physical activity ever in the evenings. Commit to adding more activity and chart your progress.

Choosing a healthy diet

In the old days, nobody thought about diets. They ate till they filled up, enjoyed the pleasure, and then loosened a belt notch to leave room for dessert. Nowadays, people still eat too much, but more often than not a fight persists within the mind. Demons duke it out for our attention. Words such as *calories, fat*, and *carbs* constantly leave one confused and filled with guilt. You can be rescued from this tumultuous torture and still enjoy many palatable pleasures. Choosing a healthy diet can be both satisfying and good for you at the same time. Discover how you can make friends with healthy food choices. Devour the information in Chapter 19.

Discovering a Mental and Physical Plan

This may in fact be one of the most make-it-or-break-it components of the ten minute tone-ups. Discovering a mental and physical plan can make the difference between winning results or just another futile attempt to tone-up. Many body builders and personal trainers believe that the mind is responsible for at least 40 percent of their success. Others believe that percentage is even higher. Most fitness programs fail because they leave out the power of the mind over body. Imagine how much better your body can respond if you mentally focus as you tone-up. Empower yourself! See Chapter 2 for more.

Chapter 2

Devising a 30-Day, Ten Minute Plan of Action

*T*his is an exciting chapter because in it I explain how you can do something positive for yourself. Schedule ten minutes of fitness a day for 30 days, and I can help you overcome all the obstacles — but you have to work with me. Getting and staying motivated can make the difference between a workout program that succeeds and one that fizzles. You decide what is your motivating kick-start. It could be an upcoming wedding, reunion, or more importantly just because you care about yourself. With the information in this chapter, you can set fast and realistic goals. No false promises.

It begins with your getting naked — in the privacy of your own home, of course. You can discover your body type and how that affects your results. To get you going on the right path, I provide a baseline fitness test, and you can use the results to create personal goals. To make this program work requires a commitment on your part. Therefore, I provide a ten minute tone-up contract that you can sign to solidify your plan. Toning up is a challenge, and this chapter can set you on the right track, but only if you accept that challenge and commit to achieving it. Are you ready? Action!

Getting Motivated

One of the biggest hurdles in most fitness programs is getting started. If there is even one tater tot of a couch potato in you, it's time to mash it. Following are some great suggestions that can help you get motivated to move. Get off that sofa. This spud's for you.

- ✔ **Select a special occasion:** Sometimes it takes a special occasion to get motivated to start a fitness program. There are experts who frown on this quick-fix mentality. One can't argue that it is far better to participate in a program that produces long-term health and fitness benefits. However, if a special occasion gets you excited enough about toning up to get you started, I say try it out. My hope is that you experience so much success that you continue on a healthy lifestyle well into the future. If you don't have a particular occasion, mark your calendar for 30 days from today. Now is the best time to get started.

- ✔ **Stop the hands of time:** Searching for the fountain of youth is a popular quest for both sexes. Extreme makeovers are everywhere. Baby boomers refuse to get old. The 30s are considered the new 20s, and even people in their 20s are clinging to their youth. Try though you may, you can't stop your chronological years from rolling along. Studies show, however, that by living a healthy lifestyle you can slow down your body age, the *physical condition* of your body, not the number of years you have lived. For example, you can be chronologically 35, but if you live a healthy lifestyle, you could possibly achieve a body age of 29. On the other hand, a 29-year-old with unhealthy habits can have a body age of 35. Using your desire to look and feel younger is a marvelous motivator. Why not strive to be your personal best at any age?

- ✔ **Change because you care:** Perhaps the best reason to begin the program is because you care about yourself. Taking care of yourself through a healthy lifestyle can lead to positive change and a sense of self respect. Changing often comes with roadblocks. By being prepared, you can avoid any detours (see Chapter 22 for ten common motivational pitfalls).

Staying Motivated

Getting and staying motivated are two different animals. How many times have you enthusiastically started a fitness program only to quit just as quickly as you started? In this section, I discuss several helpful hints to keep you jazzed about toning up and give you tips to stick to the plan.

Embracing the power of positive visualization

Devising a 30-day ten minute plan of action can only succeed if you maintain the right attitude. Being able to use that frame of thought to visualize a positive end result is very powerful. This is probably not entirely new advice. But it is information we all need to remind ourselves. Human nature often makes it easy to slip into a mode of self-deprecating behavior. Squash any negativity and focus fiercely not only on your 30-day target date, but on your daily achievable steps. By embracing a positive vision, you can make it happen.

Take a few minutes each day to think and visualize what you can look and feel like in 30 days. Now concentrate on what your specific fitness goal is for today. I find it helps to close my eyes in deep thought so that I can center in on my plan of action. When I open my eyes, I am driven to take that specific goal and accomplish it. You, too, can open your eyes to all the positive possibilities.

Creating a mental and physical plan

Enhance your ability to stick to your ten minute tone-ups by creating a mental and physical plan. This process is called mind-body fitness. Traditionally, mind-body fitness refers to exercise with an inward reflection. It stems from Eastern practices such as Tai-Chi and yoga that have permeated the West. The emphasis is on the process rather than the goal. I propose a plan that incorporates both the end result and the process. Let's face it, you have a 30-day target date. Why not enjoy the journey and still reach your goals?

Use your mind over your body to plan your long-term as well as daily goals. Use that same mind-body concentration when you flex a muscle. For example, as you work your bicep muscle, focus in the moment with an eye on your future. When you squeeze, think of your bicep as being beautiful or strong in its present state. This practice can help you enjoy the journey.

Overcoming setbacks

It's bound to happen — the setback. Something causes you to skip a workout or indulge in a midnight craving. Rather than wasting time and energy feeling guilty, you can use the temporary slip up to motivate you to a fantastic finish — a lifetime of health and fitness (see Chapter 22 for more on pitfalls).

Rewarding yourself

One tried-and-true method that can help you stay motivated is to reward yourself. It may seem a bit childish, but it works. Select something that is special to you. For example, if you stick with the program, you might arrange for a massage or take a day off work just for you. I know a guy that puts $50 in a sealed envelope and only opens it after 30 tone-up days. You can spend the reward anyway you like. Little daily rewards are also nice. Treat yourself to a bubble bath or a movie.

Be careful not to reward yourself with negative behavior. A large piece of chocolate cake is not a good choice for a reward.

Setting Fast and Realistic Goals

Nothing is more disappointing than buying into some fitness gizmo or program that costs a lot of bucks and ends up stashed in a corner, leaving you back at square one. Forget false promises, here are the steps to set fast and realistic goals.

Loving your naked self — yes, really!

The best-kept secret to setting fast and successful workout goals is to love yourself before you begin. Try this tip: In the privacy of your own home, stand buck naked in front of a mirror. Study yourself from head to toe. Rather than pick apart negative characteristics, embrace the positive: soft skin, broad shoulders, long legs, whatever you like about you. Discover what you can and can't change and go forward. Nobody is perfect. All you need to do is visit a nude beach to see that the world is filled with a wide variety of shapes and sizes — or so I've heard.

Discovering how body type affects your results

In order to set fast and realistic goals, you need to consider genetics. Each of us is born with a body type. There are three basic ones: ectomorph, endomorph, and mesomorph. You probably fit primarily into one of these, but have traits from others as well. Not one type is better than the other. I show you how to play up your strong features and give you tips to enhance the areas that you want to improve. Understanding this concept can help you become your personal best. This is the cool part, because you can have fun discovering which body type or combination of types you are. Use my recommendations to help you set realistic goals.

Endomorph

Most people are a mix of the different body types. So, if you're primarily an endomorph (read on and you'll find out), I give you the lowdown on being an endomorph in the following bulleted list:

✔ **Understanding your qualities:** If you are an endomorph, you probably have been called curvy, round, voluptuous, or shapely. Another term that both men and women can relate to is pear shaped — famous examples are Jennifer Lopez and Jason Alexander. If you are a female, you probably carry fat in your hips, legs, and butt. Endomorph men tend to have excess fat in the abdomen area. The classic endomorph has a bone structure that is often a small or medium frame. Limbs are short compared to the rest of the body, and muscle tissue has a tendency to be on the soft side.

✔ **Reaching your goals:** If you are an endomorph, you need to know that you can achieve a dynamite, toned-up shape. Because you probably carry excess fat, it may take a little more effort than other body types, but if motivated, you can do it. Do not expect to develop a super-thin model shape, because that's not realistic for your body type. Remember that good-looking bodies come in all different sizes and shapes. Start by figuring out your body-fat percentage (I explain how later in this chapter) and make healthy food choices (see Chapter 19). Because your excess weight is most likely in your stomach or lower body, be sure to exercise those areas to tone-up the underlying muscles (see Chapters 9 through 12 for lower body moves and 13 through 16 for the core). Doing aerobics is critical for an endomorph because excess fat can be a problem (there are lots of fun cardio workout choices in Chapter 20 to burn off all over body fat).

Mesomorph

Most people are a blend of body types. However, if you are primarily a mesomorph (see the bullet below to figure that out), the following information can show you what you can and cannot do to be your personal best:

✔ **Understanding your qualities:** If you are a mesomorph, you probably have an athletic build. Your muscles are quick to tone up and increase strength. The shape most often associated with a classic mesomorph is a full-length rectangular frame. You probably have large bones and muscles.

Because your chest and shoulders tend to be strong and well developed, your waist often looks smaller — a definite plus. Famous mesomorphs are Anna Kournikova and Vin Diesel.

✔ **Reaching your goals:** As a mesomorph, you have the ability to create amazing strength and definition. Lucky you, because you can quickly tone up. However, don't gloat too much because you also can rapidly gain excess fat. This is common with aging mesomorphs who don't remain active and instead pack on the pounds. Are you an undercover mesomorph? It's never too late to emerge into your top toned-up form. Be sure to include a cardio workout in your plan of action (see Chapter 20 for details). Mesomorphs tend to favor weight work over aerobics, so select a cardio activity that you enjoy doing to help you adhere to the program. Choosing healthy food choices can help speed up your results (see Chapter 19). You have the potential to cut your muscles into a shape most people only dream of. Take advantage of this genetic plus. In the next 30 days, you can begin to tone up for a lifetime (select any of the fun fitness menus in Chapter 17 and 18).

Ectomorph

Most people are not solely one body type but a blend. The following information determines whether you are primarily an ectomorph, and, if you are, how you can best reach your goals:

✔ **Understanding your qualities:** If you are an ectomorph, you are probably long, tall, and lean. A lot of people envy you because you can eat with great gusto and not gain a pound. Usually ectomorphs have very little fat, small muscle mass, and slim hips and pelvis. Ectomorphs shine in cardiovascular activities. You often have long limbs and excel in flexibility. This is a big plus, because as you age, your flexibility can help you avoid injuries. Classic ectomorphs are Cameron Diaz and Brad Pitt.

✔ **Reaching your goals:** Before you close this book thinking that you are home free in fitness, consider this: I have worked with famous actors and models who were already slim when starting my program. They discovered that being healthy is much more than being thin. If you are an ectomorph, take extra care to eat right (see Chapter 19 for helpful nutrition information). Because you probably have very little body fat, you probably avoid resistance training. Take advantage of your lean quality and focus on your 30-day tone-up goals to get ultimate results. (select fun, fast-fitness menus in Chapter 17 and full-course fitness menus in Chapter 18). Because your body responds naturally to and favors aerobic activity enjoy incorporating a cardio workout in your program. This can accelerate your tone up results (see Chapter 19 for some fun cardio choices).

Body type blends

If you read through all the body types that I describe in this chapter, you can probably find traits of yours in more than one type. That's normal, because as I point out most people are a blend of body types. That's what makes us unique. For example if your muscles are strong like a mesomorph, yet your bones are ectomorph small, you are a meso-ecto. If your waist is a curvy endomorph shape, but your shoulders are strong and broad like that of a mesomorph, you can be classified as an endo-meso. Remember: No one is perfect.

Checking out muscle fiber makeup

There are lots of genetic reasons why some people respond faster to a work-out than others. Volumes have been written on the subject. To save you some time, I briefly explain muscle fiber makeup. Understanding your muscle fiber makeup can help you appreciate why your tone-up results are so personal and individual. That way you can set realistic goals. Muscle fibers consist of the following two types:

- ✔ **Slow-twitch fibers** are for slow muscle contraction. Aerobic activities such as jogging or running incorporate these fibers.

- ✔ **Fast-twitch fibers** are for fast muscle contraction. These fibers spring into action for activities that are not aerobic, such as weightlifting.

I know it can be confusing. Just remember that fast aerobic activities require slow twitch fibers, and slow powerful activities require fast twitch fibers. The average person has a mix of slow and fast twitch fibers. Athletes are usually not as balanced in fiber makeup. For example, a professional long-distance runner probably has a higher percentage of slow twitch fibers, whereas a power lifter has a higher percentage of fast twitch fibers. There can even be variances in an individual's muscle groups. For example, your legs can be naturally stronger than your arms. That just means you have more fast-twitch fibers in your lower body than on top. This is all very normal.

You can use this valuable information to chart out fast, attainable goals. Studies show that even though you can't change a genetic muscle fiber type, you can change the way it responds. For example, if your abs are made up primarily of fast-twitch fibers, and you have minimum body fat, you can shoot for a quick six-pack. If they are made up of slow-twitch fibers, a sleek, lean, toned-up stomach is more realistic. The exciting part is you can get positive results whatever your genetic make-up. Be patient and don't compare yourself to anyone else.

Testing Your Fitness Level

The thought of taking a test may cause you to sweat. Chill out! The only sweat this test can cause is the one you get from a good workout. Ideally, it's nice to be tested by a professional at a reputable fitness center. That way, you can get a report featuring a detailed analysis of your results. For this program, I've provided a simple test that you can do in the privacy of your home. The beauty of these tests is that you don't have to compete with anyone else — it's all about you! Use it as a baseline to define your goals and individualized plan of action. For example, if you discover that your BMI is in the overweight category, you can devise a plan of action that incorporates a lot of cardio activity (see Chapter 20). If you lack strength in one or more body parts, take advantage of the prepackaged menus in Chapters 17 and 18 or mix and match them. The stretching moves in Chapter 4 are a godsend to anyone who lacks pretzel-like capability.

Focus on using this baseline as a benchmark for improvement. Repeat the tests in two weeks to chart your progress and see whether you need to shift your goals. At the end of 30 days, repeat the test again to see how far you have come along.

Body fat composition

Body fat composition is the percentage of body fat that you have relative to your muscle mass. Simply put: How "fat" are you? Body fat composition is far more important than any number on the scale, because the scale doesn't separate the weight of your bones and muscles from your fat. That's why when beginner exercisers tone up, they often see a slight weight gain. Body fat composition is a better indicator of your health.

There are several methods of testing body fat composition. Some are costly and require expensive equipment. Others are best done by a trained professional. A simple one that is free and you can do on your own is called the Body Mass Index or BMI. It's a number that comes from your height and weight. That number determines what your weight status is, ranging from underweight to obese. A BMI between 18.5 to 24.9 is healthy; however, if your BMI is 18.5 or below, you're considered underweight, and, if your BMI is 25 or higher, it is considered a health risk. (A BMI of 25 to 29.9 is considered overweight while a BMI of 30 or more is considered obese.)

Calculating your BMI

1. **Take your body weight and divide by 2.2.** For example: 150 lbs. / 2.2 = 68.18.

2. **Take your height in inches and divide it by 39.4.** For example: 5' 10" is 70 inches / 39.4 = 1.77.

3. **Multiply your answer from step 2 by itself.** For example: $(1.77)^2 = 3.14$.

4. **Divide the number from Step 1 by the number from Step 3.** For example: 68.18 / 3.14 = 21.71. The BMI is 21.71, which is in the healthy range.

You can use your BMI number as a guideline for weight loss. However, do not let that figure cause you to despair. Use this as a jumpstart for healthy, gradual, and safe weight loss. Studies show that even a small percentage of weight loss can affect the way you look and feel. Now, that's a fast and achievable 30-day goal.

Strength

There is no fancy schmancy terminology for the strength test. It basically asks how strong are you? I provide a test for upper body, lower body, and abdominal strength.

Abdominal strength

A good indicator of abdominal strength is the crunch test. For a complete description of how to do the crunch in correct form, see Chapter 15. Count how many crunches you can do using proper technique.

This is a baseline test to help you set personal goals. Do not compare with others.

Upper-body strength

You can't beat the classic push-up as an indicator of upper-body strength. Test to see how many push-ups you can do in a row without losing proper form. There are a number of push-up modifications. Select the one that meets your level of difficulty in Chapter 5.

Use the results of this test as a personal baseline as you progress through the program.

Lower-body strength

You can test your lower-body strength by doing the squats I describe in Chapter 11. Repeat as many as you can in good form. If you have exercised before, use handheld weights down at your sides. If you are a beginner, you can initiate the move with your hands on your hips.

This test serves as a baseline to chart your progress.

Flexibility

How flexible are you? A test for flexibility measures how far and how easily you can move a joint. I provide two flexibility tests: the sit and reach test and the arm and shoulder stretch test. Lack of flexibility may not cause any serious illness, but lack of mobility as you age can be frustrating and perhaps cramp an active lifestyle.

These tests provide a baseline for you to set personal goals. Do not compete with anyone else.

Sit and reach test

The sit and reach test measures the flexibility of the muscles in your back and in the backs of your legs. Even the pros use this test over expensive equipment. Simply sit up tall on the floor. Your legs should be straight out in front of you and your feet flexed up toward the ceiling. Slowly stretch forward without bouncing as you reach to touch your toes. Hold for 10 to 30 seconds. Try to repeat this stretch four or five times. If it is difficult for you to reach your toes, this indicates lack of flexibility. You can choose to do the stretching moves in Chapter 4 to increase your mobility. It helps to do this test regularly.

To increase your distance on this stretch, lift up from hips to lengthen the spine. By elongating your back, you can increase the length of the stretch by an inch or more — resulting in instant increased flexibility.

Arm and shoulder stretch test

This stretch tests the flexibility of your arms and shoulders. No fancy equipment required here. Take one hand and put it on the back of your neck. Turn your other arm around so that your palm is facing outward between your shoulder blades. Try to touch the fingers together. The closer you get the hands together, the more flexible you are in the shoulder and arm area. Repeat on the other side.

Do not arch your back to avoid any spine problems (see Chapter 1 for posture patrol pointers).

Cardiovascular fitness

An inexpensive method of measuring the fitness level of your heart is the walk test. All you need is a watch with a second hand and one mile to walk on a course or a treadmill (either is fine). Warm up for 5 minutes by walking slowly and then walk a mile as quickly as you can. Shortly before you end your walk, take your pulse (I explain how to take your pulse in Chapter 20). Record how long it took you to get to the finish line. About a minute after completing the walk, check your pulse again. This is your recovery heart rate. Try repeating this test as you progress throughout the program to see how much faster you can complete the mile as well as recover.

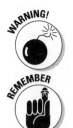

Go at your own safe pace. If a mile is too long, do only half a mile or even just a short stroll. If you can't carry on a normal conversation while walking, stop the exercise. Always start and end your walk slowly.

This test is merely a baseline. Do not compete with anyone but yourself.

Using the Tone-Up Contract

Use the contract in Figure 2-1 as a tool to help you reach your goals. With 30 days before your special event or target date, this contract helps keep you focused and dedicated. I'm with you all the way.

Making a commitment

Making your plan of action work takes commitment. Now is a perfect time to make a positive change in your life. You can do it! Read through the ten minute tone-ups contract in this chapter and take it to heart — well, at least till your 30-day target date and hopefully beyond.

Make a date, schedule ten minutes a day for yourself for 30 days. Pencil in the time — you can always change the time if you need to. Try your best not to cancel. If you are serious about devising a plan of action that gets results, make a ten-minute daily appointment with yourself. This serves as a reminder of the discipline you must maintain to achieve your dreams. (For other great scheduling tips, flip through the pages of Chapter 23 for ten ways to fit tone-ups into your schedule.)

Signing and sending to Cyndi

Some people get better fitness results if they sign a formal document. The ten minute tone-ups contract in Figure 2-1 provides a perfect compliment to your plan of action. At the start of your program, photocopy this contract and sign and date the contract. Be sure to solidify your determination by writing down your specific goals in the space provided.

To save you time and to encourage exercise adherence, I've provided space for each day of your workout. Simply check off each time you complete your ten minute tone-ups.

On day 30 repeat the fitness tests in this chapter and fill out the form. Feel free to mail or fax the form to me with your comments (contact info given at bottom of contract). I would love to hear how you are progressing. Let me know if you would like to receive more information. Good Luck!

Ten Minute Tone-Ups For Dummies
Commitment Contract

I commit to being my personal best through the *Ten Minute Tone-Ups For Dummies* program. I have dedicated 30 days to achieving my kick-start goals with the intention of carrying this new balanced lifestyle into a future of total wellness.   In the spaces provided below, I will check off each day I complete my ten minute tone-ups.

Signature _____   Start Date _____
Name (Print) _____   Phone _____
Address _____   Email _____
_____   Age _____
_____   Goals _____
Comments _____
_____

Day1 — Day6 — Day11— Day16 — Day21 —Day26 —
Day2 — Day7 — Day12— Day17 — Day22 —Day27 —
Day3 — Day8 — Day13— Day18 — Day23 —Day28 —
Day4 — Day9 — Day14— Day19 — Day24 —Day29 —
Day5 — Day10— Day15— Day20 — Day25 —Day3☺—

After completing your 30-day program, please mail, fax, or email this form in. I'd love to hear how *Ten-Minute Tone-Ups For Dummies* has worked for you. Send to:

Cyndi Targosz

STARGLOW Prods., Inc. 22647 Ventura Blvd. #502 Woodland Hills, CA 91364
Fax: (818) 888-0540 Email: Cyndi@starglowonline.com
www.STARGLOW.com

Check here to receive more of Cyndi's Secrets _____   2004 STARGLOW Prods. Inc

Figure 2-1:
Sign this
contract
and send it
in to Cyndi.

Balancing Your Plan of Action

Have you ever seen a tightrope walker at the circus? How do they walk that rope with confidence and the greatest of ease? In a word — balance. Adding balance into your life can accelerate your immediate fitness goals and, to an even greater degree, your overall well being. As you devise your plan of action for your ten minute tone-ups, think about how you can also balance your life plan. By balancing your life plan, you are less likely to fall off that rope.

It takes a developed mind, body, and spirit to maintain stability. If just one part wobbles, your entire alignment can go off kilter. This is not always easy to practice. Even as a lifestyle expert, I constantly have to remind myself of the importance of balance. One night I was writing late (my favorite time because it's quiet), and the words would not flow. I was tired after giving a presentation all day, working out, and doing the usual life stuff we all have to do. Writing about health was the last thing I wanted to do. I got so frustrated that I imagined myself as a stereotypical writer, smoking heavily and knocking back shots of whiskey. This made me laugh, because I do not smoke, barely drink, and that is not my personality at all. Guess my humor gets a little silly in the wee hours. Just before midnight, Cyndirella turned into a pumpkin. I put down my pen and reminded myself that I needed time for me. On this rare occasion, I poured myself a small glass of wine. Slowly sipping, I watched a chick flick and enjoyed my indulgent tears during this simple pleasure. The next day I was a dynamo.

Nowadays, we all are running so short of time. I've developed a way for you to balance your life and to get the most out of your ten minute tone-ups and fitness. I call the program the M.B.S. System (Mind, Body, Spirit). It's used by all my employees and clients. This system can help you think, look, and feel better as you enjoy the journey to your goals. Here then are the three components necessary for a balanced lifestyle that you can incorporate into your plan of action:

- **Mind:** Keep mentally alert. I always say that I am only as good as my last bit of knowledge. The desire to learn can keep you sharp, active, and focused. Keeping focused can take you to your tone-up goals at a faster pace. I discuss this earlier in the chapter (see the section "Creating a mental and physical plan").

- **Body:** Love yourself enough to take care of your body inside and out. Health and good looks go far beyond the image in the mirror. Embrace the benefits ten minute tone-ups can bring to your body now and into the future. (Review "Loving your naked self — yes, really!" earlier in the chapter.)

✔ **Spirit:** This is a very important part of a balanced life. It's a very personal segment that each of us experiences in a way that meets our own needs. For some, the spirit revolves around a religious conviction, whereas for others it is strictly a power within. It could even be a combination of the two. One word that applies to most people is "Attitude." Whatever your individual beliefs, one thing is certain — take your individual spirit to soaring heights, and you can achieve not only your ten minute tone-up goals, but go far beyond.

Chapter 3

Preparing for Your Workout

· ·

· ·

*P*reparing for any task is just as important as the activity itself. Imagine baking a cake without having the necessary ingredients at your disposal. The cake would be a flop. When you were a kid, did you ever have to give a speech in front of the class after not doing your homework? Two minutes in front of the classroom can seem like a lifetime of humiliation when you are not prepared. Ten minute tone-ups are no different.

In this chapter, I show you how to save time and succeed by preparing properly. I give you a list of the minimal equipment needed to get fast-fitness results. I explain all the necessary workout terms in simple language with no mumbo-jumbo and minimal jargon. I help you decide where to exercise. With the right fitness wardrobe and workout music tips, you can look cool and move to your own beat. Preparing yourself leads to a workout that can't flop and makes you rise to the top for any occasion.

Figuring out What Equipment You Need

One of the big advantages of ten minute tone-ups is that it requires minimal equipment. In fact, many of the exercises can be done anywhere, as denoted by the Anytime Anywhere icon. Following is a list of the equipment needed. They are readily available at most sporting good stores. Don't worry – just in case you are strapped for cash I also provide inexpensive alternatives.

Hitting the floor — with a mat

Several of the stretches and all of the floor work can be done on a floor mat. Some mats are ¾ inch thick, some are thinner. "Sticky" mats have a one-sided surface that clings to the floor to avoid slipping and are sold as yoga accessories. Regardless of what type of mat you select, just make sure that it's comfortable.

For an inexpensive alternative, spread out a regular towel or you can even use the carpet.

Getting smart about dumbbells

There's nothing dumb about dumbbells. In fact, using them is pretty intelligent. These weights consist of a short bar with a weight on each end. They can be round or hexagonal in shape (to prevent rolling around out of control). Dumbbells are sold in pairs and made out of several different materials.

If possible, purchase a full set. Women starting out should acquire weights of 2, 3, 5, 8, 10, 12, and 15 pounds. Men starting out should purchase weights that weigh 8, 10, 12, 15, 20, 25, and 30 pounds. If you feel your 30-day commitment doesn't warrant buying seven sets of dumbbells, try to at least buy or borrow two sets of different weights to achieve the fastest tone-up results. They cost around $1 or $2 a pound.

Objects from home can be used as an inexpensive alternative. For example, soup cans or water bottles work fine.

Buying a workout bench

A bench is a good investment if you are serious about toning up. Get one that is adjustable so that you can use it in a flat or inclined position to work your muscles at varying angles. Check out the doohickey pin that holds the incline in place to make sure it's secure and easy to adjust. Try the bench out for size before buying. I once had a client who was very enthusiastic about a bench he saw at a dirt cheap price. Fortunately, he asked me to help him with his selection. I had him get into a flat bench position at the store. You should have seen his face when his head dropped back off the bench — he was over six feet tall, and the bench was too small. Benches range from $150 to $700. Brands I like include Paramount, Hoist, and Icarian.

Try looking in your local classified section, or on eBay (www.ebay.com) or Yahoo! Auctions (http://auctions.shopping.yahoo.com) — plenty of people buy benches in that first flush of excitement and then discard them when they fall off their routine (for shame!). If a workout bench is not affordable, you can use a step bench, which I describe later in this chapter. You can also use a stool that is long and high enough for your body to rest safely and comfortably. The floor can work for many of the moves, but be mindful that it does decrease the level of difficulty.

Picking up a barbell

A barbell is a long bar, with removable weights that slide onto each end, that generally requires two hands to lift. You have seen the classic muscle man pose where the body builder is holding a barbell over his head. Barbells themselves sell for about $1 or $2 a pound, and the weights are extra. For the purpose of the ten minute tone-ups, one barbell is enough. You can invest in more as you progress.

Barbells are called *bars,* and the weights that attach to the ends are called *plates.* The clip that holds the plate on the bar is called a *collar.*

A broomstick works as an inexpensive alternative to the barbell. To increase the weight, simply attach gallon water jugs that have handles. The handles can easily slip over the broomstick. You can adjust the amount of weight by filling them with water or sand. Place them a third of the way down from each end of the broom to help keep them secure. If they're too close to the end, they may slip off.

Stepping up with a step bench

The step bench can be used in a number of ways. In appearance it resembles a miniature workout bench only it is smaller and inches away from the ground. Although this bench primarily aids you in mimicking the up and down step movements of climbing and descending stairs, it often substitutes as a workout bench. Use it flat or prop it up to an inclined positionSeveral models are on the market, selling from $15 to $100. I love the one by Reebok called the Reebok Deck. It has an adjustable incline built in. The Reebok Deck is available from www.freemotionfitness.com.

If you don't have a step bench, a raised platform will do. Just be sure that it is sturdy and at a height that is comfortable for you. You can even use the first step on your staircase for some of the moves.

Rockin' out with exercise bands

No, there aren't special musical groups specifically catering to fitness enthusiasts (although I do talk about some great workout music later in this chapter). The bands I'm referring to are made out of latex rubber, perfect for toning up quickly. They are inexpensive (about $10), offer resistance, and travel easy. These stretching pieces come in different styles and are usually color coded by the manufacturers to determine the resistance level. Some bands are flat and wide, which makes them great for exercises such as the Great Legs Band Stretch in Chapter 10. Other bands are tubular with nifty handles to make them easier to maneuver. They can be used to work every muscle group. There are even some circular ones that wrap neatly around the ankles for leg and butt exercises.

Spri makes several exercise bands to meet your individual needs. Its customer service is very helpful. Call the company at (800) 222-7774 or go to the Web site at www.spriproducts.com.

Always grip bands securely to avoid any accidental rubber-band shooting mishaps. Ouch! Also check to see if there are any holes or tears in the bands. If there are, replace them immediately.

Getting a Grip on Terminology

When starting your ten minute tone-ups, you should get a handle on the terminology. That way you can be prepared as you go through the program. Besides, your friends will be impressed when you toss the following lingo at the next social function:

- ✔ **Aerobic:** A workout that uses oxygen. For example, running.
- ✔ **Anaerobic:** The word means "not needing oxygen." It refers to short-term, high-intensity exercises that depend on stored fuel for movement. For example, weightlifting or sprinting.
- ✔ **Barbell:** A long bar with weighted plates that slip onto each end.
- ✔ **Body composition:** The percentage of body fat that you have relative to your muscle mass.
- ✔ **Cardiovascular:** The use of the heart to move large muscle groups over a sustained period of time.
- ✔ **Core strength:** Working the abdominal and lower-back muscles.
- ✔ **Dumbbells:** Short bars with permanent weighted plates attached at each end. They usually are sold in pairs.

 ✔ **Elongate the spine:** To lengthen the spine for better postural alignment (for example, standing straight).

 ✔ **Fast twitch fibers:** A muscle fiber that contracts at a fast speed, most often associated with activities that are anaerobic. For example sprinting.

 ✔ **Free weights:** Weights that are not attached to any other exercise equipment (for example, barbells and dumbbells).

 ✔ **Grip:** The way you hold the dumbbells, overhand, underhand, or neutral (palms facing each other).

 ✔ **Isometric contraction:** When a muscle contracts not changing in length.

 ✔ **Metabolism rate:** The rate at which the body breaks down food into energy.

 ✔ **Pectorals (pecs):** The chest muscles.

 ✔ **Repetitions (reps):** How many times you do an exercise (for example, ten wall push-ups are ten reps).

 ✔ **Resistance training:** When an opposite force such as a weight or gravity is used to strengthen muscles.

 ✔ **Set:** A group of repetitions (for example, three sets of ten reps).

 ✔ **Stability ball:** A ball used to improve balance and tone muscles.

 ✔ **Static stretching:** A stretch that is slow and controlled and takes a muscle through its full range of motion.

 ✔ **Tendonitis:** An inflammation of the tendon.

 ✔ **Vertebrae:** The bones of the spine.

Knowing What to Wear

Who cares what you wear? Looks don't matter. Ah, who are you kidding? Anyone who wants to tone up in 30 days probably has a healthy amount of vanity lurking within. I've got some great tips for workout wear that is very functional but looks cool, too. (Be sure to also check out my favorite workout-wear manufacturers in Chapter 24.)

Searching for shoes

Athletic shoes are one workout item you don't want to buy based on looks. Search for your sole mate — a pair you can be comfortable with and know is the right fit. Start by understanding your own feet. Are they flat? Wide? Do they roll outward or inward from the ankles. If you said yes to any of these questions, you probably need a good arch support. It helps to share your foot needs with a knowledgeable sales rep. Fortunately, there are a number of excellent shoe manufacturers (I mention several in Chapter 24). In addition to fit, look for stability, flexibility, and shock absorption. That just means you can jump up and down and side to side without discomfort. I actually jump and run in the store before I buy. Some places let you live with the shoes for a while before you make a full commitment. Make sure you only walk on the carpet. You can't return them used. There are even some retail establishments that have you run outside before you buy. Experts watch to see how you wear your shoes so that they can fit you in the appropriate pair.

Just a foot note: Do not exercise in old, beat-up shoes. They offer no support and can cause injury.

Putting your spandex on — one leg at a time

Many experts recommend wearing baggy workout clothes, yet they themselves prance around in skimpy spandex. Don't get me wrong — you can wear baggy clothes if that is truly your personality. However, all too often both men and women dress in t-shirts and sweats that fit them like a tent. If that's you, be honest with yourself — what are you trying to hide? If you dislike your body, review "Loving your naked self — yes, really!" in Chapter 2. With 30 days to your target date, baggy clothes can give you a little too much room to grow. Instead of sloppy, opt for slightly loose-fitting clothes that are attractive yet comfortable. Snug clothes are fine, too, as long as you can move. I actually prefer snug but comfortable clothes because they serve as a constant reminder of where I want my weight. Plus, in snug clothes, you can watch your muscles work when you're toning up!

The key word is *fit*. It doesn't matter whether you are big, small, tall, wide, or thin, as long as your workout wear fits (see Chapter 24 for suggested workout wear manufacturers).

Workout wear is very personal. Nobody should dictate to you what your style is. Be confident in the body you have been given as you strive to be your best.

Following are some great workout-wear words of wisdom:

- ✔ **Layer your clothes:** Your body temperature changes as you work out. Layering your clothes can help you adjust to the temperature.

- ✔ **Take it to the streets:** Nowadays you can find clothes that easily go from your workout to the streets. Everyday active wear can help you bend and stretch anywhere and everywhere for faster results. I live in mine.

✔ **De-emphasize a large butt:** Wear dark pants with a loose-fitting but not too baggy top. Avoid pockets on your behind that draw attention to your rear end.

✔ **Play up your parts:** Decide what your attributes are and play them up. If you are a guy with a great chest, a muscle tank shirt might suit you. A woman with nice legs — short shorts.

✔ **Choose quality fabric:** Workout wear can take quite a beating from all the use. Choose fabric that is made to last. I like supplex because it can survive several washings, absorbs perspiration, and moves easily with my body. Cotton is nice in the summer when the weather is warm. It is quick to soak up sweat.

✔ **Downplay negatives:** Everybody has features that are less than perfect. Downplay those with a little fashion savvy. For example, if you are a guy with a beer belly, a super-tight waistband is not going to hold it in. The proper fit can make you look your best. If your arms flap in the wind, avoid sleeveless tops. A top-heavy woman should not wear super-tight tank-tops.

Going for gloves

Novices hardly ever use workout gloves. Yet gloves are handy fitness items. Wearing them can make you feel like a pro. If you intend to use weights of any type, gloves can enhance your workout. I find that gloves help with my grip on the weights. If your hands sweat, gloves can help you avoid any slippery accidents. Wearing gloves also helps prevent unsightly calluses, which is pretty important when you shake hands at a special occasion. The best gloves are usually made from natural fibers. They need to fit snugly but comfortably. Be sure that they protect your knuckles and cover the top of your fingers. I like the ones that have padding in the palm area, usually made out of fabric or filled with gel. A few good brands of gloves are Champion and Harbinger.

Studies have shown that the equipment at public gyms are breeding grounds for germs, but if that is your place to tone up, don't stop now. Using workout gloves can protect you from picking up unwanted bacteria on your hands.

Finding the Right Place to Exercise

I'm often asked: Where is the best place to exercise? The beauty about the ten minute tone-ups is they can be done nearly anywhere. Whether you select the gym, your home, or while traveling, it works. Decide what suits your needs and stick to the program.

Sizing up your home gyms

There are a lot of reasons to do the ten minute tone-ups at home. If you're on a tight schedule, nowhere is more conveniently located than your home, and the hours are perfect. Unlike most gyms, at home you are free to open and close your workout area whenever you like. Use the time alone to become comfortable with your own body. Sometimes being around other fitness enthusiasts can be a little intimidating (though in reality, they are usually too busy worrying about their *own* insecurities to think about yours — everybody has their "stuff," you know). Nevertheless, sometimes home alone workouts can do wonders to increase your self confidence (see "Loving your naked self — yes, really!" in Chapter 2). If a home workout is for you, then go ahead and hang up that "Open sign" on your door.

Here are some pointers to design a perfect home gym:

- ✔ **Find your ten minute tone-up corner:** Every home exerciser needs a designated workout area. Whether it's the foot of your bed, the spare bedroom, or the guest house outside your mansion, it needs to be your personal ten minute tone-up corner. Psychologically, this can help you to feel like saying, "Okay, it's time to go to the gym."

- ✔ **Define your needs:** When setting up a home gym, make sure you define your needs. For reaching your goals with ten minute tone-ups, very little space or equipment is needed. On the other hand, if you decide to build from there, you may require more equipment and space. Being prepared means you have a clear vision of where you are now, where you are going, and what you have to do to get there (review the power of visualization in Chapter 2).

- ✔ **Buy home equipment:** Minimal equipment is required to do the ten minute tone-ups. Ideally, you need dumbbells, a workout bench, some resistance bands, and not much more. See "Figuring out What Home Equipment You Need" earlier in this chapter. I also offer inexpensive alternatives.

- ✔ **Purchase a multigym:** A multigym has several exercise stations built into one piece of equipment. This is not necessary for the ten minute tone-up program, but it can certainly enhance your workout. They usually run upwards of $1,000 for a good one. Try out each station to make sure it's comfortable. Check for stability — a flimsy one won't last, and then you are less likely to use it. Some good brands are Paramount, Hoist, and Universal. Most sports specialty stores carry a wide variety.

Several retail places such as "Play It Again Sports" sell used sporting goods. You can find stuff in good condition at a great price.

Joining a health club

If you are the type of person who is most motivated to work out around other people, joining a gym is for you. You can easily take a fast-fitness menu from Chapters 17 and 18 with you. Choosing a gym for your personal needs can be a bit more complicated. Some cities don't offer a lot of choices, whereas others seem to have one on every corner. Whether it's a hoity-toity spa facility or a transformed auto garage shop with fitness equipment doesn't matter. What's important is that you feel comfortable and you use it.

Here are some pointers to help you decide what health club to join:

- ✔ **Location! Location! Location!:** Location is pretty self-explanatory. If you are not near the gym, you are less likely to use it. Consider where you work. It's possible that a location near your office may be more convenient than near your home. Stop in after work, do your workout, leave refreshed, and possibly miss all the traffic.

- ✔ **Cost:** Consider your budget. If you are stressing about making payments, the health benefits are lessened. Invest in one that suits your checkbook. Prices range from $300 to $3,000 a year. Calculate benefits in your cost. For example, if childcare is included, you can save money in the long run.

  Just because a gym is cheap doesn't mean that it's no good, nor is an expensive one necessarily good. Try a one-week free trial to size it up.

- ✔ **Question the staff:** Are they friendly? Knowledgeable? It helps to have a prepared list of questions so you don't forget anything.

- ✔ **Question the members:** The best way to find out the real scoop on a gym is to talk to the current members. They usually love to gossip to potential members. Locker rooms are great for this camaraderie.

- ✔ **Try out the equipment:** Make sure you are comfortable using the equipment. Check out the quality. If most of the pieces are draped with "Out of order" signs, that's not a good sign.

- ✔ **Check limitations:** Several gyms limit the time you spend on equipment, or they limit towels, hours, and so on. Be sure that your gym doesn't require too many limitations.

- ✔ **Rate the cleanliness:** Gyms are breeding grounds for germs. Make sure the place is kept up. Check the locker rooms, showers, and rest rooms. Do they regularly wipe down the equipment and vacuum?

Traveling

If traveling plans happen to fall before your 30-day target date, no need to despair. You can prepare to do your ten minute tone-ups on the road. Simply take along this book or take one or more of the fast-fitness menus in Chapters 17 and 18, and you're good to go. Throw bands in your bag for resistance — they're described earlier in this chapter (for more great traveling fit tips, see Chapter 21).

Increasing Weight Safely

As you progress through the ten minute tone-ups, you can expect your muscles to shape up and get stronger in the process. Periodically check your progress with the strength test in Chapter 2. It serves as an indicator for when to increase the weight you are using. Certainly bumping up the weight is a new accomplishment to reach a new level in fitness. However, you have to know how to increase the weight safely.

Several different training systems can be used to get maximum results with weights. To name a few, there's the single set system, which is 1 set of 8 to 12 repetitions, and the multiple-set system, which is 3 to 6 sets of 8 to 12 repetitions.

Another system is circuit toning, which is 1 set of 8 to 20 repetitions and is further described in Chapter 17. Several other systems have been devised, but the preceding are the least you need to know for this program. After each exercise, I tell you your training system options.

Most exercise sets in this program require one to three sets of eight to ten repetitions. Once you are able to accomplish all of your sets in 12 repetitions using good form without fatigue, you are ready to increase the weight. Do so in small increments of approximately 2 to 5 pounds.

To check whether you are ready to increase the weight used in an exercise, be sure that you can perform the move using the correct form described. If your form is off, you may actually need to use less weight to avoid injury.

Choosing Music to Move and Motivate You

When preparing for your workout consider choosing your favorite music to move and motivate you. Research confirms that music affects your mind, body, and spirit. It has been proven that physiological changes actually occur within your body during music. It can help to create a rush within you that catapults you to your ten minute tone-ups goals.

In addition to feeling good, new research shows a relationship between music, exercise, and brain alertness. Working out with music may improve the way your brain functions, though certainly more studies are needed. But for now, enjoy listening to motivating music as you exercise. Do your ten minute tone-ups with music before a college exam or an important office meeting — it may improve your performance.

Some music is specifically designed for working out. That's what many pros use. Most consumers don't know about this, but here's the inside scoop: Choosing music that is specifically designed for a workout can improve your performance and reduce the risk of injury. Let me explain. When you work out to regular CDs, they may motivate you, but it's too easy to "cheat" when there's a break between songs or when a slower song is playing.

To avoid injury, select music with appropriate BPM (beats per minute). BPM is important because if your music is too fast, you could hurt yourself, and if it's too slow, you won't get as effective of a workout.

Follow these guidelines:

- **120-135 BPM:** Toning up and beginner cardio.
- **Up to 126 BPM:** Step aerobics.
- **Up to 145 BPM:** Walking, jogging, intense cardio.

You can figure out the BPM of your favorite music. Listen for the music's main beat and count the beats per minute as you snap your fingers.

Several manufacturers have done all the work for you. You can purchase workout CDs that come in a wide range of styles to suit your taste. No need to worry about BPM — that's done for you, too. Following are some of my favorite workout music manufacturers and their contact information:

- **Muscle Mixes:** 800-52-MIXES (64937); www.musclemixes.com
- **Power Music:** 800-777-BEAT (2328); www.powermusic.com
- **Dynamix Music:** 800-843-6499; www.dynamixmusic.com

Chapter 4

Warming Up and Stretching

. . . .

In This Chapter

▶ Discovering best results through warming up and stretching

▶ Stretching your upper body

▶ Getting your lower body stretched out

▶ Making sure your abs and lower back get a good stretch

▶ Checking out rejuvenating moves

. . . .

*T*hrowing a log on the fire and lifting your legs up on a cushy ottoman while knocking back a shot of brandy is one way to warm up and give yourself a stretch. However, with only 30 days to target your trouble spots, the best fire to admire is the one within your belly that motivates you to get off the couch!

In this chapter, I explain the importance of including an aerobic warm-up and stretching moves in your workout. The stretches I provide perfectly complement your ten minute tone-ups. They're safe, effective, and should never be eliminated. Your body works more efficiently and speeds up results when you include a good warm-up and some stretching in your exercise routine, so keep reading to get on track to better results.

Warming up and Stretching for Best Results

Whenever you do your ten minute tone-ups, always include an aerobic warm-up and stretching moves. Both keep your muscles in a safe and healthy state. Many people try to leave them out of the workout — don't! By not doing these moves, your muscles remain stiff and cold and therefore more prone to injury. Suddenly, a simple exercise can become dangerous.

Getting in your aerobic warm-up

Whenever you start your ten minute tone-ups, including an aerobic warm-up gets the circulation moving throughout your body. *Aerobic* means that you are using oxygen to complete the exercise, so, basically, you'd better keep breathing. Warming up can be compared to starting up that old car in the morning in the dead of winter or waiting for your computer to go through its complete cycle of booting up. Try to use a car or computer before it's warmed up, and you'll get nowhere. Same goes for your body.

Your body can perform its best in a minimum amount of time if your muscles have been warmed up with an aerobic activity. Here's the secret: Select something that you enjoy doing that uses oxygen to get your heart rate up, such as walking, running, or jumping. Perform the activity for a minimum of three to five minutes to get your circulation going. Never skip this (unless you're skipping, of course).

Choose an activity that uses muscles close to the body part you are targeting. For example, if you plan on toning your biceps and triceps, try swinging your arms while walking.

To really speed up the process of reaching your goals, turn your aerobic warm-up into a full-blown cardiovascular workout. (Chapter 20 cites several examples that can help you reduce fat while you increase your endurance.)

Always start and end your aerobic warm-up activity at a safe pace. A good measure of this is that you should be able to carry on a comfortable conversation throughout.

Stretching for success

When to stretch has become a controversy among experts (see the sidebar, "Stretching the issue"). To maximize results, you should stretch your muscles after your ten minute tone-ups when they are warm from working out. Stretching lengthens your muscles and improves their flexibility. Stuff you do every day is much easier when your muscles and joints are flexible. Think of reaching for the top shelf, grabbing a child ready to fall, or lifting yourself up from a slip on the ice. So, after a workout — just keep stretching by following these stretching tips:

🖊 **Hold each stretch.** You should hold each stretch for a minimum of 10 to 30 seconds.

🖊 **Be sure to stretch the area you are working on.** For example, if you are doing ten minute tone-ups for the legs, stretching your lower body is a priority. Of course stretch your entire body for the best results.

🖊 **Stretch daily.** It's best to stretch every day, but if you can't fit that into your schedule try to stretch a minimum of twice a week.

🖊 **Avoid stretching a cold muscle.** Begin each stretching session with at least three to five minutes of an aerobic warm-up (for example, run, jump, skip, dance). This gets the blood circulating and prepares your muscles for the work they are about to do.

🖊 **Avoid bouncing while stretching.** It is better to hold the stretch for the recommended 10 to 30 seconds. This is called *static stretching*. During the holding position, you can adapt your body to your personal level of difficulty. That just means to stretch as far as is comfortable without causing pain.

🖊 **Breathe.** Do not hold your breath. Use slow deep breaths to help you chill out and to facilitate the movement. Take a deep breath to inhale at the start of the stretch and then exhale as you hold the stretch. Keep breathing deeply throughout the move.

🖊 **Use stretching as a wonderful way to relax.** The more you do it, the better you feel.

🖊 **Keep on stretching.** Don't give up. If you are new to stretching, the moves may make you feel a little stiff. You may wonder how any one could ever find it pleasurable. As you progress, your muscles can loosen up, and your flexibility can improve. Be patient.

Stretching the issue

Stretching, believe it or not, is a controversial issue in the fitness world. It fuels much debate. Recent research shows that stretching before a workout does little to lower the risk of injury. These studies indicate that muscle injury might have more to do with lack of muscle strength, overuse, or bad training. These experts promote stretching at the end of a workout. On the opposite end of the spectrum are professionals who feel stretching should occur before an activity. For example, they think you should stretch the shoulders before playing golf or stretch the hamstrings before running. Before you say, "Forget about it!" consider the consensus. On balance, most experts still agree that to reach your tone-up goals, stretching (before and/or after) is a necessary element of a good workout program.

Stretching Your Upper Body

Stretching can enhance your upper-body workout. (See Chapters 5 through 8 for powerful and effective upper-body exercises.) Do the following stretches after your upper-body workout for the safest and fastest results:

Neck Stretch

This very simple move is extremely effective. Not only does it serve as a perfect upper-body stretch for the neck and shoulders, it does wonders to relax your muscles. Throughout the day, it's not uncommon to catch me doing a neck stretch to help minimize any upper-body tension that may have accumulated.

Taking slow deep breaths will help to relieve any muscle tightness and better prepare your upper body for the exercises that you do.

Getting set

Stand tall with your shoulders relaxed but not slouched.

Hold your abs in tight and butt tucked under. Do not arch your back. Practice proper posture during this relaxing stretch. (Chapter 1 is filled with excellent posture pointers you can use during your upper-body stretches.)

The stretch

Gently bring your head toward your right shoulder. Hold it there for 10 to 30 seconds (see Figure 4-1). Keep the shoulders relaxed. Repeat on the other side.

Shoulder Rolls

This move is perfect to do throughout the day as well as after your upper-body workout. It stretches the neck, back, and shoulders and helps to improve posture.

Avoid doing shoulder rolls at a fast and jerky rate. If you deliver the move that I describe in an extremely slow and controlled manner, you can achieve fast, safe, and effective results. Always stop if you feel pain or are prone to neck and shoulder injuries. (See Chapter 1 for more on knowing your medical limitations.)

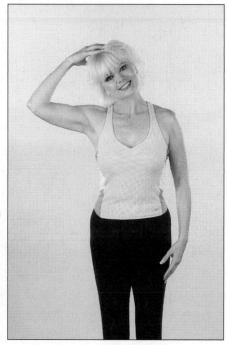

Figure 4-1:
The Neck
Stretch
reduces
neck and
shoulder
tension.

Getting set

You can stand or sit for this move — you can even try it during work breaks at your computer. Place your hands on your hips.

Hold your head up high as if it was being pulled with a string from the top of your head. Tighten your abs. Keep the neck relaxed.

The stretch

Shoulder rolls are done in the following two parts:

- ✔ **Backward rolls:** In one slow but fluid motion, lift your shoulders up toward your ears, bring them back and down in a circular motion as you squeeze your shoulder blades together and gently take them down and around to the front. Do this slow fluid and continuous motion ten times (see Figure 4-2A).

- ✔ **Forward rolls:** In one slow but fluid motion, lift your shoulders up toward your ears. Round the shoulders and gently bring them forward and then down in a circular motion in the direction of your back and up again. Do this slow, fluid, and continuous motion ten times (see Figure 4-2B).

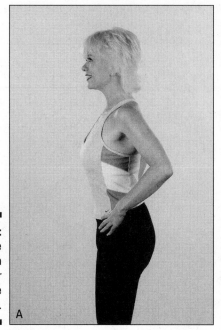 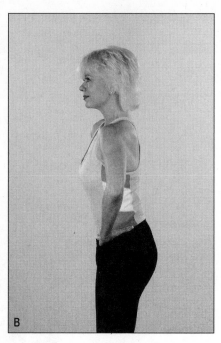

Figure 4-2:
Improve
posture with
Shoulder
Rolls done
slowly.

A   B

Upward, Backward, Forward Reach

This move stretches the entire upper body. Use it to stretch your chest, arms, and upper back and shoulder muscles.

Getting set

Stand tall and erect with your feet hip-width apart. Hold your abs in tight and butt tucked under. Keep your head up high and shoulders relaxed.

The stretch

The entire exercise is done in three parts — upward reach, backward reach, and forward reach:

- ✔ **Upward reach:** Clasp your fingers together as you lift your arms up over your head so that your palms are facing up toward the ceiling. Stretch up toward the ceiling. Hold the stretch for a minimum of 10 to 30 seconds (see Figure 4-3A), and then return to the getting-set position.

- ✔ **Backward reach:** With your arms down and toward the back, clasp your fingers behind you. Keeping your elbows straight, squeeze your shoulder blades together and push your shoulders as far back as it is comfortable. Hold the stretch for a minimum of 10 to 30 seconds (see Figure 4-3B), and then return to the getting-set position.

The higher you raise your arms behind you the more advanced the move, but maintain proper posture — do not arch your back — throughout the move.

✔ **Forward reach:** Clasp your fingers as you take your arms straight out in front of you at shoulder level. Keep your elbows straight and palms facing the wall in front of you. Round your shoulders as you stretch and reach forward. Hold for a minimum of 10 to 30 seconds (see Figure 4-3C).

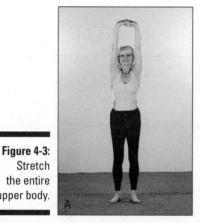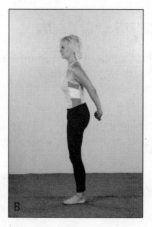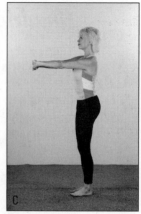

Figure 4-3:
Stretch the entire upper body.

Stretching Your Lower Body

I understand that a hectic schedule may prevent you from wanting to stretch your lower body. Don't cheat yourself. The following lower-body stretches can enhance your workout. (See Chapters 9 through 12 for excellent lower-body exercises to go along with these stretches.)

Hip and Groin Stretch

This move simply cannot be done enough. It stretches your hip and groin area with an emphasis on the hip flexors. The hip flexors are the muscles opposite your butt muscles. (See Chapter 11 for a detailed description of how stretching them can enhance your lower-body workout.)

Getting set

Start from a standing position.

The stretch

Lunge forward so that one leg is in front of the other. Your front knee should be bent in a 90-degree angle so that it is lined up directly over your front foot and ankle. Bend forward from your waist as you support your weight by both hands on the floor. The back leg should remain straight but do not lock your knee. Press your hips toward the floor (see Figure 4-4). Hold the stretch for a minimum of 10 to 30 seconds. Repeat on the other side.

Quadriceps Stretch

This is a stretch I've incorporated into my everyday life. It stretches the quads, and is actually kind of fun.

Getting set

Start from a standing position, you can use a chair or the wall for support. (See Chapter 1 for proper posture pointers.)

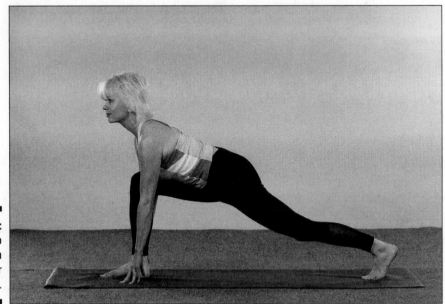

Figure 4-4:
Include hip
flexion
in your
program.

The stretch

Rest your left hand on the back of a chair or the wall for support. Take the right hand and lift your right ankle up as if you were kicking your butt with your heel. Both knees should be next to each other, and your hips should be forward (see Figure 4-5). Hold the stretch for a minimum of 10 to 30 seconds. Repeat on the opposite side.

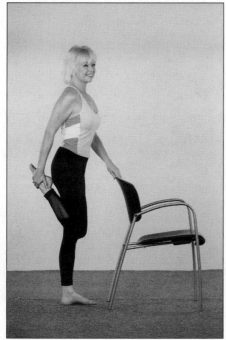

Figure 4-5: Do the Quadriceps Stretch during a coffee break.

Hamstring Stretch

Use this stretch to enhance your lower-body workout and to increase flexibility. It targets the hams (your hamstring muscles — not cheesy show-offs).

Getting set

Lie on your back with knees bent and feet flat on the floor.

The stretch

Lift one leg straight up. Without raising your hips off the floor, use your hands to stretch the hamstrings toward you (see Figure 4-6). Hold the stretch for a minimum of 10 to 30 seconds. Repeat on the opposite side.

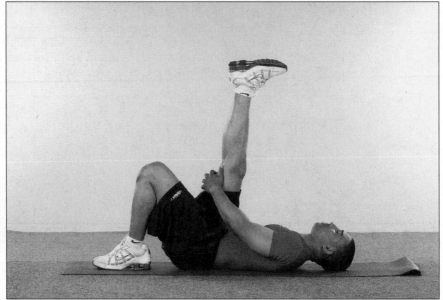

Figure 4-6:
The
Hamstring
Stretch
enhances
flexibility.

Calf Stretch

Stretching your calves will help you have a little extra spring in your step — a result of increased flexibility. (This move also complements the calf exercises in Chapter 12.)

Getting set

Start from a standing position.

The stretch

This movement is two parts. Using a chair or a wall for support, place one leg behind the other:

- ✔ **Work the gastrocnemius:** Bend the front knee slightly while you keep the back leg straight and heel down. Lean your hips forward to stretch the back calf (see Figure 4-7A).

- ✔ **Work the soleus:** Bend both knees with heels down. Lean your hips forward to stretch the back of the calf (see Figure 4-7B).

Hold each stretch for a minimum of 10 to 30 seconds. Repeat on the opposite side.

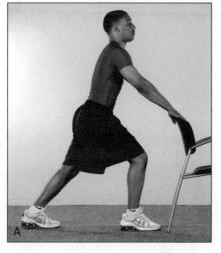 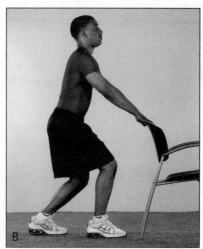

Figure 4-7:
The Calf
Stretch
wakes up
tired legs.

Stretching Your Core: Abs and Lower Back

The center of your body that acts as the foundation of your stability and balance — the *core* — includes the abs and lower back. (See Chapters 13 through 16 for core strength and toning exercises.) Do the following stretches after your core workout to enhance the results.

Standing Abs

Get to know your abs with the Standing Abs move. It stretches the whole core area.

Getting set

Stand tall with your feet hip-width apart. Lift your arms straight up toward the ceiling with your palms facing forward (see Figure 4-8A).

The stretch

Using slow, controlled movements, bring your arms down to your sides. Your palms should end up facing inward. At the same time, round your back, bring your chin to your chest, and contract (squeeze) your abdominal muscles (see Figure 4-8B). Hold for ten seconds. Return to start. Repeat ten times.

Exhale when you contract or squeeze the abdominals. Inhale when you return to start.

Concentrate on contracting your stomach muscles rather than using your hips or arms for the movement.

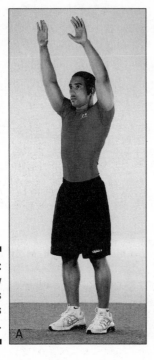

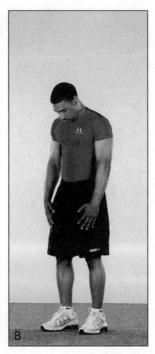

Figure 4-8:
Get to know your abs with this move.

Cat Stretch

I love the Cat Stretch. You may think it's because I have a feline nature, am a Leo, and my initials are C.A.T. However, it just plain feels really good when you do it. The Cat Stretch focuses on your abs and lower back.

Getting set

Kneel on all fours (see Figure 4-9A).

Keep your back flat. Head and neck should be aligned with your spine so that your vertebrae are elongated. (See Chapter 1 for proper posture details.) Do not drop your head at the start.

The stretch

Slowly contract and squeeze your abs in toward your spine as you drop your head gently and round your back (see Figure 4-9B). Pause for a moment and slowly return to the starting position. Told you it feels good! That is one repetition, and it should last 20 seconds. Repeat three times or more if you like it like I do.

Inhale at the start of this stretch so that your stomach actually pouches out to let the air in. Exhale slowly as you contract your abs to round your back.

Figure 4-9:
The Cat
Stretch
feels really
good!

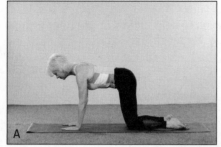 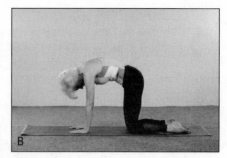

Rejuvenating Your Mind and Body

Stretching exercises can do more than increase your flexibility. They serve as a psychological spark that rejuvenates your mind and body. Doing these moves not only relaxes your body, but calms the mind, too. Take time to do the stretches with an inward reflection, and your motivation to reach your goals can skyrocket. (Chapter 2 further discusses the benefits of creating a mental and physical plan.) Try these following rejuvenating stretches.

Cobra

This traditional yoga move may appear snakelike, but it's really a charmer. It stretches the chest and abs, elongates the spine, and strengthens the buns and thighs.

Getting set

Lie outstretched on your stomach with your legs straight behind you. Rest your forehead on the floor. Place your palms to the side so that your fingers are pointing forward and slightly to the front of your shoulders.

Bend your elbows so that they are pointing up to the ceiling. Press your hands down to lift your chest slightly off the floor (see Figure 4-10A).

The stretch

Press your hands even harder into the floor as you begin to straighten your arms to help lift your upper torso. Stretch only as far as it is comfortable. Hold for a minimum of ten seconds (see Figure 4-10B). Repeat.

Press your hip bones into the floor throughout the stretch. This will help with stability.

If you have wrist problems, do not press off the palms. It is safer to push off the forearms. Include your arms to help lift your upper body. Keep your lower body stable to avoid back injury.

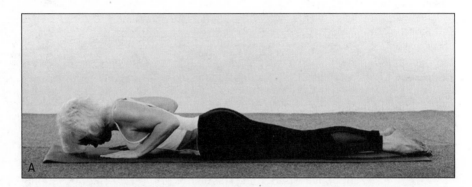

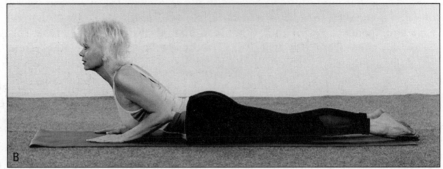

Figure 4-10:
The Cobra is a traditional yoga move.

Child Pose

The Child Pose takes you back to the womb for a feeling of inner peace and tranquility. This popular yoga move stretches the entire spine as it relieves tension. Yoga teachers frequently call upon it whenever their students need to regroup from moves that are too challenging. You can use it as your personal center — far away from hectic everyday stuff.

Getting set

Kneel on the floor so that your heels are resting on your buns.

The stretch

From your hips, bend forward until your forehead touches the floor. Elongate the spine but don't tense it up. Rest your chest on your thighs; your arms should lie gently along your side (see Figure 4-11).

Slowly and deliberately inhale and exhale. Feel your breath expanding and relaxing your rib cage.

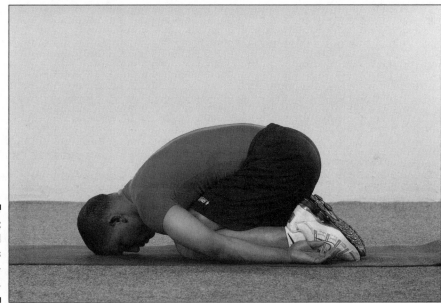

Figure 4-11: The Child Pose is rejuvenating.

If you are stiff, place a pillow under your ankles to assist with the stretch. Many of my male clients who lack flexibility use this modification.

Try the Child Pose with arms stretched in front of you and palms up for a little more challenging, but still very rejuvenating, stretch.

Part II
Upper-Body Workouts

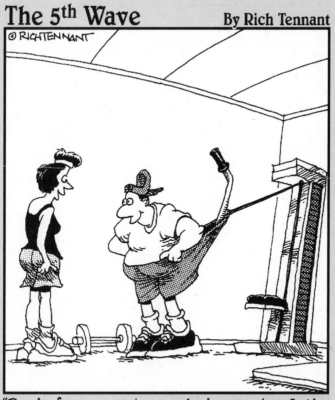

The 5th Wave   By Rich Tennant

"Ready for our next upper body exercise? Let's continue with the brain."

In this part . . .

I designed this compilation of exercises to tone the upper torso. Do these exercises if you want to target your chest, upper back, shoulders, or arms. I discuss some basic anatomy and provide some great tips on technique so you know exactly what you're working on and how best to work it.

Chapter 5

Shaping a Tip Top: Chest

In This Chapter

▶ Being up front about your chest muscles

▶ Discovering top technique tips

▶ Strengthening and defining the chest

Your chest muscles enable a number of practical, everyday movements that you probably take for granted. Pushing a cart in the grocery store, for example, or hugging a dear friend would be impossible without the chest muscles. Every time you use a pushing or hugging action, your chest muscles are activated.

Of course, sculpted chest muscles make you look good, too. Strutting your stuff is easy when you have strong, defined chest muscles. Traditionally, men have flexed their chest muscles in an effort to appear pumped, and the exercises in this chapter show men how to achieve that sculpted shape. Women, on the other hand, often shy away from chest exercises for fear of either ending up looking like a guy or decreasing their breast size. Rest assured ladies, these tone-ups will *not* make you look like a guy. In fact, strong, firm chest muscles actually provide support for and uplift your breasts. Healthy, toned chest muscles make you feel more confident making your entrance in a strapless dress, swimsuit, or any other clothes. (For more chest exercises specifically for women, get a copy of my upper body workout video tape "Best Bust" at www.starglow.com).

For health reasons, you should keep your chest muscles in shape because they're attached to and often work with your shoulder joint, which is very prone to injury. Strong chest muscles make for a healthier shoulder joint. (For more on the shoulder joint, see Chapter 7.)

Getting to Know Your Chest Muscles

You can achieve results in less time if you understand how your chest muscles work. This basic anatomical information focuses your mind on the physical movement of the chest. (Refer back to Chapter 1 to learn how creating a physical and mental plan can help you achieve better chest results.)

If you can visualize your chest muscles and feel their exact point of contraction, you will know exactly where to squeeze or exert force on your chest during an upper body exercise.

The scientific term for the chest muscles is the *pectorals.* You have probably heard the slang term *pecs.* I use both of these interchangeably. If you talk about pecs, you'll sound like a pro. The pectoral muscles are the fan-shaped muscles of the chest. Figure 5-1 highlights the following muscles of the chest:

- ✔ The ***pectoralis major*** runs diagonally from your collarbone to the top of your arm.

- ✔ The ***pectoralis minor*** reaches from the breastbone to the upper arm.

They work in conjunction with the shoulder and arm muscles for pushing and hugging actions. Because the pectoral muscles form such a large muscle group, it is not unusual to think of them in terms of upper, lower, and mid-chest level. The type of chest movement that you perform determines which of those muscle fiber levels are stimulated.

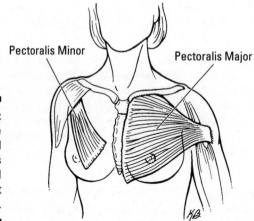

Pectoralis Minor

Pectoralis Major

Figure 5-1:
These are
the pectoral
muscles
developed
in chest
exercises.

Chest Exercise Techniques

Use the following techniques when doing chest exercises so you can achieve safe, fast results:

- ✔ **Warm-up and stretch:** Always include an aerobic warm-up at the beginning and stretch at the end of your chest workout. Refer to Chapter 4 for a detailed description of how to incorporate stretching moves into your chest routine.

- ✔ **Use the proper equipment:** Some of these exercises will require an adjustable home workout bench as well as a set of dumbbells. (Refer to

Chapter 3 for more on this equipment, which can be found at any sporting goods store.) You can also substitute a step bench, a stool, or if a bench is unaffordable, use the floor. Soup cans or water bottles work great as weights, too.

✔ **Breathe correctly:** Breathing properly during a chest exercise accelerates positive results. Be sure to exhale during the point of exertion. Simply put — exhale or blow the air out during the "pushing" part of the exercises in this chapter. For example, when doing the flat bench press, inhale at the start and exhale as you push the weight away.

✔ **Do a practice set first:** Weighted chest exercises always work best if you complete one set with minimal or no weight before you do the move with heavier weight. This practice set serves as a warm up before each individual chest exercise and is not to be confused with the more general chest workout warm up explained in Chapter 4.

✔ **Adjust the bench angle:** You can personalize your chest workout by adjusting the angle of the bench. Doing so shifts the focal point of where the chest muscles are being worked. For example, using a flat bench draws attention to the middle chest area, but using a bench that is on an incline works the upper chest muscles. A bench that is in a decline position (with your head angled down) works the lower chest muscles. Working the lower chest muscles is less critical because those fibers cover a smaller area of the chest.

✔ **Keep your elbows bent:** Don't lock your elbows during chest exercises. Doing these exercises with straight arms can put unnecessary stress on your elbow joint and cause an injury such as tendonitis.

✔ **Don't arch your back:** Arching your back during a chest exercise can put too much pressure on the lower spine and cause injury. If you can't keep your spine in neutral alignment, try using less weight. (See Chapter 1 for more posture pointers.)

Balancing your back and chest

Putting balance in your life makes for a healthier lifestyle, yet how easy it is to leave out the balancing act when it comes to the muscles of our body — particularly the back and chest. Keep pumping those pecs to shape a sculpted chest, but to achieve maximum results, don't skip on the back.

The back muscles are the opposite group of muscles to the pectorals. If you over-train your pecs and forget about the back muscles, you will start to take on the physique of a gorilla. You've seen the stereotypical bodybuilder with

the short neck and hunched forward body. That's usually the result of an unbalanced workout — too much chest, not enough back.

Developing chest muscles to the point where they are stronger than your back muscles equates to a body that is prone to injury. So see Chapter 6 for some great upper back exercises to complement your chest routine. Selecting the menu items in Chapter 17 or 18 for chest, upper back, and shoulders conveniently provides you with a ready-to-go, packaged upper body program with built-in upper body balance.

Isometric Chest Press

If you want your chest muscles to look great for a special event in the near future or if you just can't find the time to devote to shaping them up, you'll love this exercise. This simple but effective move works the upper, middle, and lower pectoral muscles. It's a secret exercise that several celebrities I know have been doing for a long time in their dressing rooms between TV and movie takes. Now you can do it, too.

Getting set

Start by standing with your feet planted firmly on the ground hip-width apart. Clasp your hands together in front of you.

The exercise

Do this exercise in each of the following positions:

Waist level: Bend your elbows as you clasp and press your hands together in front of you at waist level. You should feel your chest muscles flexing as you press. Hold for five seconds and release (Figure 5-2A). Repeat the movement.

Chest level: Bend your elbows as you clasp and press your hands together in front of you at chest level parallel to your nipples. Contract your chest muscles. Hold for five seconds and release (Figure 5-2B). Repeat the movement.

Shoulder level: Bend your elbows as you clasp and press your hands together in front of you at shoulder level or slightly higher. Feel your chest muscles contracting. Hold for five seconds and release (Figure 5-2C). Repeat the movement.

Other options

Cross your wrists: For a change so as not to get bored you can, do the move with one wrist crossed over the other and press them together for five seconds in each of the exercise positions. Remember to flex your chest muscles throughout the moves.

Change the order: For variety, try doing these exercises in a different order. Feel free to mix them up since order won't affect the results.

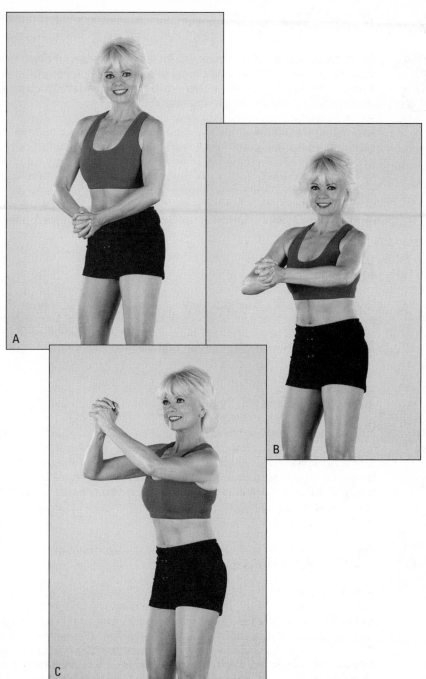

Figure 5-2:
Using these
three
positions,
you can
work the
entire chest
area
anywhere.

Wall Push-up

All levels benefit from this exercise. An advanced exerciser may need to do more repetitions than the traditional push-up before feeling fatigue. However, anyone can do a few here and there throughout the day, which adds up, feels good, and is far better than doing nothing.

Although the traditional push-up (see the section "Other options" in the next exercise) works the chest, arms, and shoulders, wall push-ups are an excellent alternative if you are a beginner and want to build up your strength to a more advanced level. They work the same muscles, but with less difficulty, and are still very effective. Wall push-ups are also a good choice if you want to strengthen the chest but have back problems because they put no stress on your spine. (See Chapter 1 for tips on how to prevent back problems.)

Getting set

Standing in front of a bare wall, lift your arms up to shoulder level. Place your palms against the wall so that they are slightly wider than your shoulders. Your fingertips should be pointing up. Back your feet a couple feet away from the wall so that your elbows are bent as you lean on an angle into the wall (Figure 5-3A).

The exercise

Inhale before beginning the exercise and exhale as you push off the wall until your arms are in an outstretched position with elbows slightly bent (Figure 5-3B). Inhale as you go back to the starting position. Repeat the move five to ten times. As you progress you can gradually work up to 20 or more wall push-ups for increased chest strength. When you are able to complete the exercise with ease using the proper form described, increase the repetitions by a few Wall Push-ups.

Hold your tummy in and tuck your butt under throughout the exercise. This helps to support your upper body.

Other options

Pause: This is an advanced variation. As you return to start from the extended arm position, stop and pause halfway. Hold for a few seconds and continue to move slightly forward. Stop and pause again for a few seconds. Stop and pause one more time before returning to start.

Use a slow pace: This is another advanced variation. Try doing the wall push-up at a very slow pace. Count very slowly up to four as you push off the wall and count slowly to four as you return to start. This increases the tension in the chest and arms.

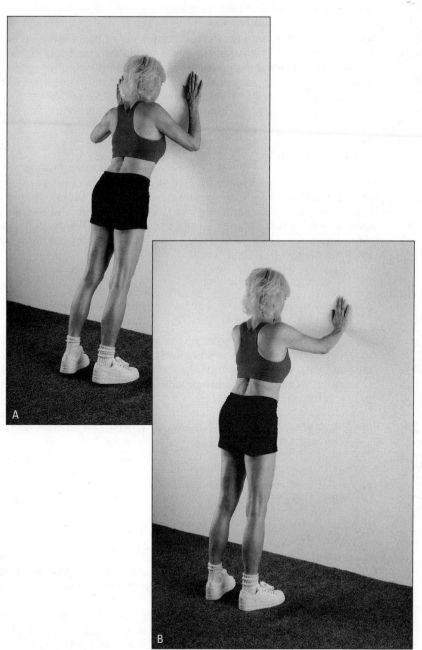

Figure 5-3:
The wall
push-up
puts no
strain on
the back.

Modified Push-up

For some people, the traditional push-up is too challenging, so the modified push-up is a better choice. The modified push-up works the entire chest area as well as the shoulders and the triceps.

Selecting a push-up that is appropriate for your fitness level increases the level of safety and yields better results. Never choose a traditional chest push-up if you cannot maintain the recommended form throughout the entire exercise. There are plenty of modifications available. For more push-up choices, see the section "Other options" after this exercise.

Getting set

Start by lying on your stomach. With your elbows bent, place your palms flat down on the floor a little above your shoulders and slightly to the side. Your fingertips should be pointing forward. With crossed ankles and bent knees, raise your body up to almost straighten your arms (Figure 5-4A). Remember not to lock your elbows. Keep your chin tucked in a few inches toward your chest but do not drop your head.

The exercise

Inhale as you slowly lower your chest till your upper arms are parallel to the floor (Figure 5-4B). Exhale as you slowly return to start. Hold your abs in tight and keep your spine in neutral alignment throughout the exercise. Repeat the movement 10 times and eventually try to do 20 modified push-ups or more for increased chest strength.

If you have knee trouble, try doing the movement on an exercise mat or carpet to give you a greater degree of comfort.

Other options

Wall push-up: I describe this easier option earlier in the chapter.

Traditional push-up: This more challenging move is the same as the modified push-up, except that your lower body is balanced on the balls of your feet (where your toes attach) rather than on your knees.

Raised feet push-up: This advanced move gives your upper chest a demanding workout. Do it the same way as the traditional push-up, but place your feet on a raised platform such as a stool or a raised step bench.

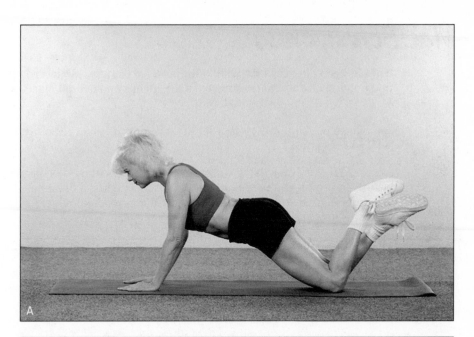

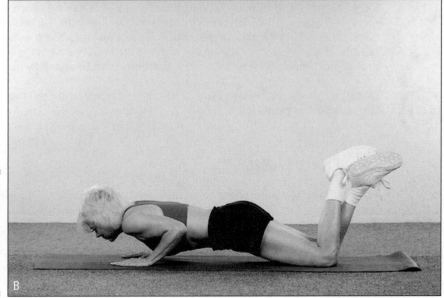

Figure 5-4:
The modified push-up is a very effective chest move.

Flat Bench Press

The flat bench press works your chest muscles with an emphasis on the middle and outer pectorals. It also stimulates the triceps and deltoid muscles.

Getting set

Lie on your back on a flat workout bench. Your feet should be firmly planted on the floor or, if you prefer, up on the bench. Holding a dumbbell in each hand, raise your arms up so that they are above your shoulders with your palms facing forward (Figure 5-5A).

Hold your tummy in and keep your spine in neutral alignment. Do not arch the back.

The exercise

Inhale as you slowly lower the dumbbells down. For safety, your elbows should end up just below your shoulders and in line with the center of the chest to avoid joint injury (Figure 5-5B). Exhale as you raise the dumbbells back to start. Do one or two sets of eight to ten repetitions. As you progress, do two or three sets of eight to ten repetitions with increased weight.

Do not lock your elbows. Keep your shoulder blades squeezed together throughout the exercise.

Other options

Use the floor: If you're prone to shoulder joint or rotator cuff injuries or need to simplify this exercise, position yourself on the floor instead of a bench. The arms stop at, instead of stretch just below, shoulder level.

Do it halfway: Bring the weights down only half way if you have a shoulder joint injury. It takes pressure off the rotator cuff. (Chapter 7 provides tips to strengthen the muscles of this gentle joint.)

Raise your feet up: Do the exercise with your feet raised up in the air. It relieves the pressure from your lower back — a real plus for people with back problems. Raising up the feet is also challenging for everybody because you must stabilize your body by contracting your abs to complete the move. This aids in strengthening your core (abs and back) while you work the chest. (For more core moves, check out Part IV.)

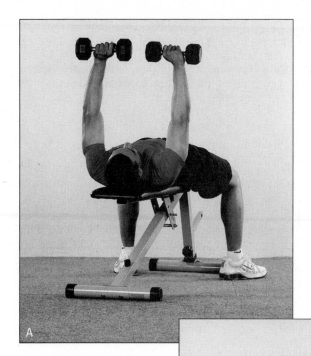

Figure 5-5:
Keep a natural curve in your back for the entire chest movement.

Incline Fly

The Incline Fly targets your pectoral muscles, particularly the fibers of the upper chest. It also stimulates the front deltoids and indirectly the triceps, which act to stabilize the move.

Getting set

Place your adjustable workout bench in an incline position at about 30 degrees.

Press your back into the incline portion of the bench while maintaining neutral alignment (see Chapter 1 for more tips on posture). Do not arch your back or flatten it. Plant your feet on the floor or the bench. Hold a dumbbell in each hand. Raise the dumbbells straight up over your chest with your palms facing each other (Figure 5-6A).

The exercise

Lower your arms in a half-circle pattern, thus keeping your elbows slightly bent and your arms still while moving from the shoulders. Stop just below shoulder level (Figure 5-6B). Hold your abdominals in and return to the starting position. Do one or two sets of eight to ten repetitions. As you progress, do two or three sets of eight to ten repetitions with increased weight.

Be sure to inhale as you open your arms up and exhale as you return to the starting position.

Focus on contracting your chest muscles as you raise the dumbbells up. To avoid injuring the rotator cuff, do not take the arms lower than just below shoulder level when you take the dumbbells down.

Other options

Use the floor: Make this chest move easier by doing it on the floor. It's not quite as effective, because the arms will not be able to open up to just below shoulder level as they do on a bench, but it does put less stress on your joints. This works the middle chest as compared to the incline position, which emphasizes the upper chest.

Do it on the decline: Place your workout bench in a declined position so that your feet and lower body can be positioned above your head. Doing a decline chest fly will stimulate fibers in your lower chest muscles. Avoid doing this exercise if you have elevated blood pressure.

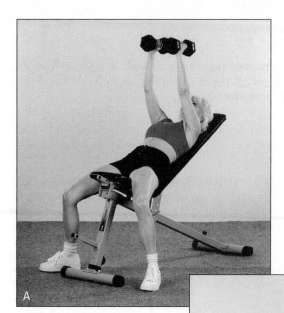

Figure 5-6:
The Incline
Fly hones
in on the
fibers of the
upper chest.

Dumbbell Pullover

The dumbbell pullover delivers a lot of bang for the buck. Not only does it strengthen the entire chest but it works the upper back, shoulders, arms, and even the abs. This chest move is a super-size value!

Getting set

Lie on your back on a flat bench with your feet planted on the floor or on the bench for comfort. Holding one dumbbell with both hands, lift your arms up above your shoulders. Your palms should be facing up toward the ceiling. One end of the weight should rest in your palms while the other end hangs down over your face (Figure 5-7A).

Hold your stomach in and keep your spine in neutral alignment. Do not arch your back, and use less weight if you can't maintain natural posture.

The exercise

Inhale as you slowly lower the dumbbell behind you until the weight is even with the back of your head. Do not bend the elbows since the move is coming from the shoulder joint. See Figure 5-7B. Exhale as you slowly return to start. Do one or two sets of eight to ten repetitions. As you progress, do two or three sets of eight to ten repetitions with increased weight.

Hold onto that weight! If you lose focus, you'll be dropping it on your face.

Other options

Use the floor: Doing the dumbbell pullover on the floor decreases the level of difficulty.

Place shoulders on bench: Try this advanced version of the dumbbell pullover. Rather than lying on the bench, keep your hips off of it with your feet planted flat on the floor hip-width apart so that your body is perpendicular to the bench. Rest only your shoulders on the bench. Hold your abs in tight to help with stability. Pull over the dumbbell to the opposite side of the bench and return to start to complete the movement. Remember not to hyperextend your spine in this challenging pullover move when the back is extended. Using too much weight can put your back in a dangerous arched position. Beginners do not try!

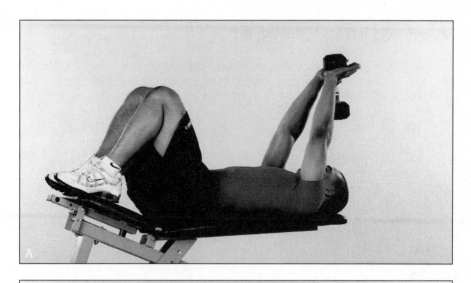

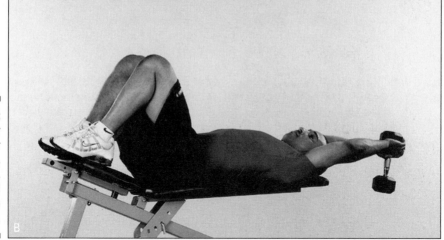

Figure 5-7:
Work your
chest, upper
back,
shoulders,
arms, and
abs in one
move.

Chapter 6

Working Out the Upper Back

In This Chapter

▶ Finding basic upper back muscles

▶ Avoiding mistakes during upper back moves

▶ Checking out upper back exercises

*W*orking on the upper back is not usually as popular as working out other body parts, such as the abs, chest, or legs, but it's just as important. A strong upper back pulls you through the day, and I mean literally pull through. Activities, such as pulling your golf clubs along the course, schlepping your luggage through an airport, and dragging your dog to the vet, use upper back action. Plus, sculpted upper back muscles present a marvelous view when you exit a room. Whether you wear a suit and tie, a low back dress, or a muscle shirt, a well-toned upper back makes your waist and hips appear smaller. Because the upper back is so connected to the shoulders, it's not uncommon to incur shoulder joint injuries, if you have a weak upper back. The shoulders end up overcompensating when doing everyday tasks without a strong upper back for support. Strengthening the back can prevent injury to the fragile shoulder joint. (For more information on the shoulder joint see Chapter 7.)

In this chapter, I show you the various muscles that make up your upper back, followed by practical workout tips and several great upper back exercises. Have fun getting your upper back into shape!

Getting to Know Your Upper Back Muscles

Studying your upper back muscles makes it easier to get positive results. I've provided an illustration that clearly shows where the muscles of the upper back are located (see Figure 6-1).

Using a handheld mirror, take a look at your own upper back muscles. Watch as you squeeze your shoulder blades together, shrug your shoulders, and move your upper back in any number of ways. Then compare your upper back muscles to the ones in Figure 6-1 so you can recognize them as they contract.

✔ **Looking at your lats:** The largest muscle group in the back is known as the *latissimus dorsi.* Gym rats call this group the *lats* — and, of course, now you can, too.

Reaching from your lower back to your upper arm bone, the lats, when developed, provide that fabulous V-shape. The lats work in combination with the arms for pulling and rowing movements. (See Figure 6-1.)

✔ **Taking a peek at your traps:** The *trapezius* reaches from the middle of your back to your shoulders and back in again. You have a pair of them, and they form the shape of a trapezoid, simply called the *traps.* If you aren't sure which muscle group is the traps, just shrug your shoulders — that uses the traps. (See Figure 6-1.)

✔ **Recognizing those rhomboids:** Between your spine and shoulder blades is a group of muscles called the rhomboids. Technically they are called the rhomboidei (don't worry, not even most experts use that term). Now that you're armed with this impressive trivia, you should know that the rhomboids are anything but trivial. Along with the traps, the rhomboids are responsible for squeezing your shoulder blades together. This squeezing action is critical to good posture, upper body balance, and avoiding shoulder joint injuries.

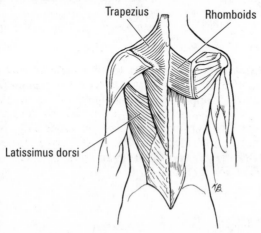

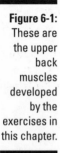

Figure 6-1: These are the upper back muscles developed by the exercises in this chapter.

Trapezius   Rhomboids

Latissimus dorsi

Upper Back Exercise Techniques

Following the upper back techniques in this chapter makes for a successful workout: Expect a great-looking back view, as well as strong and healthy upper back muscles. Follow these pointers to perfect your upper back workout:

- **Warm-up and stretch:** You must do an aerobic warm-up before and stretch after your upper back workout. (Refer to Chapter 4 for how to include stretching moves in your upper back program. Do not skip this component!)

- **Get the right equipment:** These exercises require minimal home equipment. Pick up a set of dumbbells, an adjustable workout bench, and a tubular resistance band with handles (Spri makes a good one). This equipment should be available at most sporting goods stores. (See Chapter 3 for more equipment information.) You can also use a step bench or a stool if a workout bench is not available. In a pinch, you can use soup cans or water bottles for weights.

- **Breathe properly:** As always, exhale as you use exertion, and inhale as you return to start and prepare for the next exertion.

- **Use your back not your arms:** When doing upper back exercises, the arms will naturally spring into action. Although that is normal, focus on the upper back contraction (squeezing) rather than on your arms. Think of your arms as assistants to the moves. With practice, the feeling of upper back flexion is more apparent. Flexion is just a fancy term for flexing or muscle contraction.

- **Maintain good posture:** You need to keep your spine elongated to successfully perform upper back exercises. To keep your spine elongated, imagine that a string is holding your head, neck, and spinal column like a marionette. (See Chapter 1 for more on posture.)

- **Avoid body shifting:** It's easy to be overzealous when lifting weights during an upper back exercise. Everyone wants fast results. However, lifting weights that are heavier than you can handle causes your body to shift inappropriately. You may be able to complete the move, but it is momentum that is helping you rather than the upper back, and it's not momentum that you're trying to make more attractive. Use only the amount of weight that you can handle in an upper back exercise without shifting your body out of correct form.

One-Arm Dumbbell Row

The One-Arm Dumbbell Row works the upper back and stimulates the muscles of the front upper arms and shoulders.

Although the arms are used in this exercise, the primary focus should be on your upper back muscles. Visualize and feel the upper back contractions throughout the movement. (See Chapter 2 for more on visualization.)

Getting set

Standing on the right side of a workout bench, place a dumbbell in your right hand; let it hang down next to your body with your palm facing in. Bend from your waist and rest your left hand on the bench for balance (see Figure 6-2A).

Throughout the movement: Hold your stomach in; keep your back flat, so that it's parallel to the floor; align your neck with the rest of your back; and keep your knees slightly bent.

The exercise

Using slow and controlled movements, lift the arm that is holding the weight up until your hand touches your waist and your elbow and shoulder are parallel with the floor (see Figure 6-2B). Focus on using your upper back muscles to lift the weight rather than just lifting your arm up and down. Do not rock your body during this movement. Slowly return to start. Do one or two sets of eight to ten repetitions on each side. As you progress, do two or three sets of eight to ten repetitions on each side with increased weight.

Inhale when you begin and exhale as you lift the weight up.

Other options

Decrease the weight: If you can't maintain the proper form I describe in this exercise, decrease the weight. Sometimes it is better to use no weight till you master the technique and your upper back muscles are stronger.

Rotate the elbow: For a more advanced move, place your left knee and your left hand on the bench to keep your body stable. Raise your right arm up and back until your shoulder and elbow are parallel with the floor. Take the right elbow a little higher than your back and rotate it toward your left side. Return to the start. Be sure to flex your upper back muscles. Do both sides.

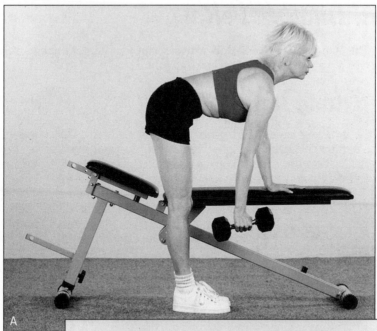

Figure 6-2:
Use slow
controlled
movements
during the
One-Arm
Dumbbell
Row.

Seated Dumbbell Row

The Seated Dumbbell Row helps to sculpt your upper back muscles.

Getting set

Sit with your knees and legs together at the end of a workout bench. Holding a dumbbell in each hand, bend from your waist until your chest rests on your thighs. Let your arms hang down so that the dumbbells are close to your feet and your palms are facing behind you (see Figure 6-3A).

The exercise

Inhale at the start of this exercise and exhale as you lift the weights up to hip level while turning the palms toward the front. Raise your elbows slightly higher and squeeze your shoulder blades together (see Figure 6-3B).

Pause and hold the squeeze for a few seconds. Slowly return to start, twisting the palms so that they are facing behind you again. Do one or two sets of eight to ten repetitions. As you progress, do two or three sets of eight to ten repetitions with increased weight.

Inhale at the start of this exercise and exhale as you lift the weights. Inhale when you return to start.

You may feel the urge to move your arms out to the side, but doing so works the shoulder rather than the upper back, and that's a completely different exercise. If you want shoulder exercises, visit Chapter 7.

Use a full range of motion during the Seated Dumbbell Row. That just means taking the exercise through a complete movement, including shoulder blade contraction in the up position to a good stretch when your arms are hanging down.

Other options

Make it easier: Don't twist your palms. Keep them facing back throughout the exercise.

Make it harder: Increase the resistance (weight). But don't increase the weight until you have mastered the proper technique I describe for the Seated Dumbbell Row.

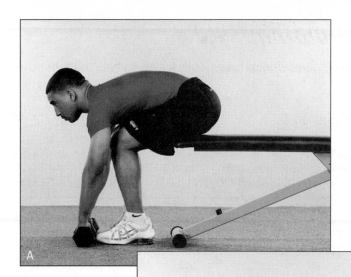

Figure 6-3:
Use a good
stretch in
the down
position and
squeeze the
shoulder
blades in
the up
position.

Kneeling Two-Arm Row

This dynamite move really defines the upper back.

Getting set

Get down on one knee as if you were making an old-fashioned marriage proposal. Bending from your waist, rest your chest on your front leg. Hold a dumbbell in each hand and stretch your arms to the floor so that your palms face in toward your body near your front foot (see Figure 6-4A).

Hold your stomach in to avoid excess stress on the back. Your abs act as a support system during this upper back move.

The exercise

Slowly raise your elbows up toward the back and inward (see Figure 6-4B).

Don't allow your chest to lift up off your knee. Using the entire upper body to assist you in the move takes the emphasis off the upper back muscles.

Squeezing your shoulder blades together, hold for a few seconds, release, and then slowly return to start. Do one or two sets of eight to ten repetitions. As you progress, do two or three sets of eight to ten repetitions with increased weight (see Figure 6-4B).

Remember to exhale as you lift the weight up and squeeze the shoulder blades together. Inhale as you return to start.

Hold your abs in tight and don't arch your back.

Other options

Sit: If you have a bad knee or are just uncomfortable kneeling, try doing this exercise while sitting on a chair. Lean forward from your waist to rest your chest on the chair and continue the move.

Increase the weight: Take this exercise to a new level by increasing the weight. Just make sure you maintain the proper form I discuss in the exercise.

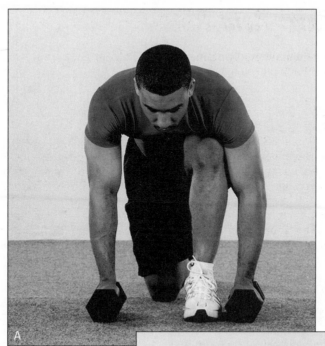

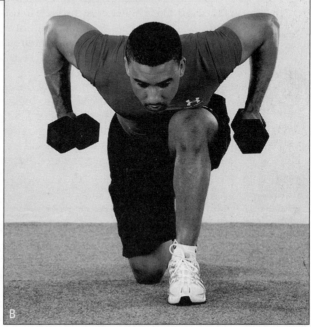

Figure 6-4:
The
Kneeling
Two-Arm
Row
delivers a
strong
upper back.

Bent Forward Row

Looking to shape up the upper back fast? The Bent Forward Row zeroes in on those upper back muscles instantly.

Getting set

Standing with your feet flat on the ground and hip-width apart, hold on to a set of weights using an underhand grip. An *underhand grip* is gym talk for grabbing the weights with your hands so that the palms are facing forward at the start of the exercise.

Keeping your low back slightly arched, bend over from the hips so that your upper body is almost parallel to the floor. Let your arms stretch down in front of you (see Figure 6-5A).

The exercise

Lift the weights straight up to your rib cage so that your elbows are pointing up (see Figure 6-5B). Return to start. Hold your body stable in the same position for the duration of the movement. Be sure to keep a slight bend in your knees. Do one or two sets of eight to ten repetitions. As you progress, work up to two or three sets of eight to ten repetitions.

Keep the elbows in toward your body throughout the movement. Taking them out to the side will work the shoulder muscles rather than the upper back — a different exercise. For a selection of a shoulder exercises, see Chapter 7.

Inhale at the start of the movement and exhale as you lift the weights up.

Other options

Intermediate Bent Forward Row: Do the same move with an *overhand grip,* which means that your palms are facing the back at the start of the exercise.

Advanced Bent Forward Row: If you are an advanced fitness enthusiast, try doing this exercise while standing on one leg and using either the overhand or underhand grip explained in the Bent Forward Row description. This version of the movement challenges your stability and coordination.

If you are a novice, do not try these intermediate and advance options!

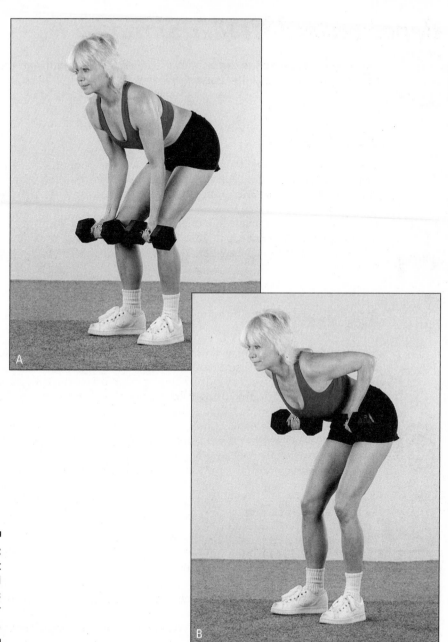

Figure 6-5:
The Bent
Forward
Row shapes
the upper
back.

Upper Back Shoulder Shrug

This timesaving exercise can be done anywhere. It very efficiently works both the trapezius muscle of the upper back as well as the shoulders. (See "Getting to Know Your Upper Back Muscles," earlier in this chapter.)

Getting set

Standing tall, hold a dumbbell in each hand with your arms down in front of you. Palms should be facing in toward your thighs.

Hold your stomach muscle in and elongate the spine as if a string were pulling you up from the top of your head. Hold your chin toward your chest and keep your knees slightly bent (see Figure 6-6A). For more on posture, visit Chapter 1.

The exercise

Lifting your shoulders up as if to say, "I don't know" activates the upper back and shoulder muscles (see Figure 6-6B).

Slowly return to start. Do 20 repetitions.

In this exercise, you need a couple of dumbbells, but if you happen to be in line at the grocery store take the advantage of the time. Use two cans of peas as a substitute for the weight.

Other options

Use no weights: This upper back exercise is even effective with no weight. Try doing it while you are waiting to download something off the Internet. For more timesaving tips, see the Anytime-Anywhere moves in Chapter 17.

Keep shrugging: For a more challenging move, hold a shrug in the upward position for several seconds. As you hold, give your shoulder blade an extra squeeze to emphasize the trapezius and rhomboids. Slowly return to start.

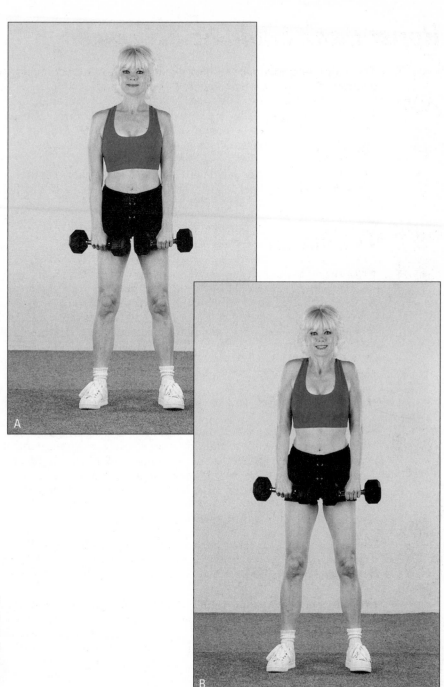

Figure 6-6:
Shrugging
activates
upper back
action.

Resistance Band Lat Pull Down

The Resistance Band Lat Pull Down works the upper back muscles as well as activates the shoulder and biceps.

If you have neck problems, are susceptible to neck injuries, or experience pain during this exercise, skip this move. (Refer to Chapter 4 for some effective upper back stretching exercises.)

Use a tubular resistance band with handles (Spri makes one that is available at sporting goods stores. Take a look at Chapter 3 for more details.)

Getting set

Standing with your feet hip-width apart, hold the two handles of the tubular resistance band in your left hand and hold the opposite end in your right hand. Keeping your elbows slightly bent, raise your arms up over your head. Your left palm should be facing in while your right palm is facing forward. Stand erect with your stomach in and butt tucked under. Do not lock the knees (see Figure 6-7A).

The exercise

Keeping your left arm stable above your head, bring your right arm down by bending your elbow out to the side — as if you were Robin Hood shooting an arrow into the sky. Stretch the band until your right elbow is pointing down and the resistance band is taut (see Figure 6-7B). Slowly return to start. Repeat the movement on the other side. Do the sequence five times.

As you pull the band down, keep the waist straight to avoid wrist injury.

Other options

Sit: Sitting provides more stability during this exercise. If you need better balance, have a seat!

Adjust the resistance: You can make the exercise easier or harder by varying the resistance. Resistance bands are available in different strengths (see Chapter 3 for more information). Any band can also be adjusted for resistance variations. Shortening the distance between your hands increases the intensity; whereas, lengthening the distance between your hands decreases it.

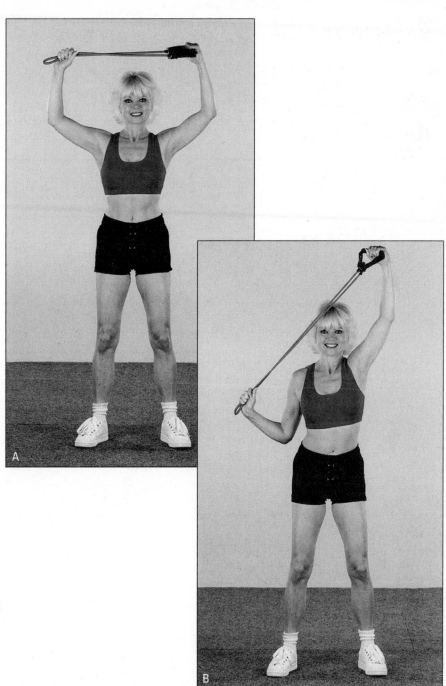

Figure 6-7:
The
Resistance
Band Lat
Pull Down is
a fun upper
back
exercise.

Give it a rest

Resting your upper back muscles enhances your results. This surprising information may be hard to believe, yet it is very true. Your upper back muscles are actually repairing themselves during your day of rest. It is during that repair time that they get stronger and firm up. Never work the upper back muscles with weights two days in a row. It is best to work them two to three days a week on alternate days. For dynamite lats, traps, and rhomboids — give it a rest.

Chapter 7

Shrugging Off Shoulder Slouch

In This Chapter

▶ Understanding your shoulder muscles

▶ Discovering great shoulder-exercise techniques

▶ Performing shoulder exercises for deltoids and rotators

*R*egardless of your weight or size, going around with droopy, slouched, or hunched shoulders can make you look ten pounds heavier. On the other hand, developing and defining your shoulders can dramatically improve your appearance. Your shoulders, in fact, are amazingly important and flexible parts of your anatomy — yet a sedentary lifestyle will heap too much stress on them. So, you should include shoulder exercises in your workout even if you have very little time. Because most people find that their shoulder muscles develop relatively quickly, even a little time spent on shoulder exercises may give you strong, sculpted shoulders, which by comparison can make your waist appear slimmer and a large derriere appear smaller.

More importantly, developing strong, healthy shoulder muscles can prevent many of the injuries caused by ordinary activities such as loading groceries, lifting children, moving furniture, or pitching a ball. The weekend warrior who engages in little physical activity during the week and then, without warming up, suddenly thinks he's Michael Jordan on Saturday is particularly susceptible to shoulder trouble. One ill-advised lay-up, for example, could put your shoulder out of commission for six months to a *year*. I've seen it happen. So, use the timesaving tone-up exercises in this chapter to do wonders for how you look *and* protect you from injury.

You use your shoulders in numerous exercises. You can't work out your back or chest muscles without incorporating your shoulders. So you can create a very effective workout by working the chest, back, and shoulder muscle groups together. For more on customizing your workout to meet your individual needs, see Chapter 17.

Getting to Know Your Shoulder Muscles

A breath mint ad once showed a bulky, retro bodybuilder grinning and posing. The caption read, "Nice Altoids." The ad, with its play on words, was alluding to the fellow's shoulders. Figure 7-1 shows what shoulder muscles look like.

Deltoid   Rotator Cuff (partial view)

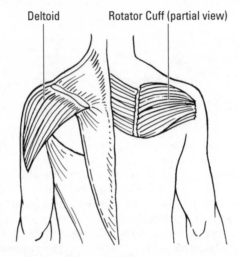

Figure 7-1:
The two types of shoulder muscles: deltoids and rotators.

✔ **Dissecting your deltoids:** *Deltoids* are what you think of when you think about shoulders — they are your main shoulder muscles. Starting near the base of your neck and running almost halfway down your upper arms, your deltoids are actually made up of the following three separate muscles that allow your arms to move in many different directions:

- The **anterior (or front) deltoid** lifts your arm straight out in front of you and up.

- The **medial (or side) deltoid** raises your arm out to the side and up.

- The **posterior (or rear) deltoid** moves your arm backward and up.

✔ **Rooting out your rotators:** Beneath the deltoids lies another group of shoulder muscles called the *rotators*. The rotator cuff allows you to twist or rotate your arms in their sockets. You couldn't change an overhead light bulb, for example, without your rotators. Called the *rotator cuff,* two muscle groups make up the rotators:

- **Internal rotators** rotate your arms inward.

- **External rotators** rotate your arms outward.

In combination, the deltoids and the rotator cuff make up the *shoulder joint,* also called the *ball and socket joint.* The shoulder joint is truly a marvel of mobility, allowing you to direct your arm in nearly any direction.

You probably get much more fired up to work your deltoids because rotator muscles are smaller and less visible — okay, invisible (except in Figure 7-1). However, you can't neglect the rotators because they are so prone to injury. That's why I've included two rotation exercises in this chapter, to make your rotator cuffs stronger. Strengthening the rotator cuff protects the whole shoulder joint.

Shoulder Exercise Techniques

You should keep the following in mind when performing shoulder exercises:

- ✔ **Get the right equipment:** For delts, you need a pair of light dumbbells. For your rotators, you need a tubular resistance band with handles (such as the one made by Spri), available for $10 or so at most sporting goods stores. (See Chapter 3 for more details on exercise equipment.)

- ✔ **Relax:** A lot of stress is carried in the shoulders, as well as in the neck.Reduce your tension by taking a deep breath before each exercise and dropping your shoulders to their natural position. Hunching your shoulders up by your ears not only creates unnecessary tension, it makes your neck look shorter. And nobody needs that.

- ✔ **Use appropriate weight:** Because you can easily damage the shoulder joint, be sure to use an appropriate weight for you. If you cannot maintain the correct form that I describe for each shoulder exercise, you are probably using weights that are too heavy. (Review Chapter 3 for details on how to increase weight safely.)

- ✔ **Breathe properly:** Many of my clients ask me about proper breathing during an exercise. To make the proper breathing technique easier to remember, I give breathing an XXX rating: eXhale on eXertion during eXercise.

- ✔ **Warm up and stretch — always:** Before you begin the exercises in this chapter, be sure to do an aerobic warm-up. Include stretching at the end of your workout. (See Chapter 4 for some great stretching moves.) The aerobic warm up will increase the circulation in your system and send more blood and oxygen to your shoulder muscles. The stretching at the end will bring down your heart rate to a safe level and enhance your flexibility. Don't leave these out!

Side Lateral Raise

This exercise works the medial deltoid muscle. It's a great way to quickly tone up your shoulders.

Getting set

Stand with your feet planted on the ground, hip-width apart. Hold a dumbbell in each hand, positioned in front of your legs. Palms should be facing each other. Hold in (contract) your abs. Lean slightly forward from your waist so that your weights are in front of your legs at every start. Do not lock your elbows. (See Figure 7-2A.)

Stand tall and maintain a natural arch in your back (see Chapter 1 for more posture tips).

The exercise

Raise the weights up and out to the side, as if you're going to start flapping your wings (see Figure 7-2B). Use slow controlled movements. Stop and pause just before your arms are parallel to the floor at shoulder height. Do not lift the weights higher than shoulder level. Slowly lower the weights to the starting position. Do one or two sets of eight to ten repetitions. As you progress you can do two or three sets of eight to ten repetitions with increased weight.

Inhale at the start of the Side Lateral Raise and exhale when you lift the dumbbells up. Inhale as you return to start.

Other options

Reduce the weight: If this exercise is too difficult, try it with less or even no weight.

Bend your elbows: For greater ease, do the exercise with your elbows bent at a 90-degree angle. Although this option is not quite as effective as the original move, it provides a safer alternative for people prone to shoulder injuries.

Sit down: For variety, try doing the exercise seated. Start with your hands down at your sides and your elbows slightly bent. Keep your feet flat on the floor and staggered to support the back. Do not raise the weights above shoulder level.

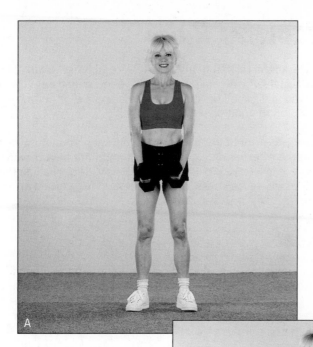

Figure 7-2:
The Side
Lateral
Raise can
give you
wider, more
defined
shoulders.

Alternating Lateral Raise

This exercise is a slight variation on the Side Lateral Raise. It also works the medial deltoid muscle. By alternating, I mean you're only using one dumbbell at a time, which means you'll be slightly off-balance, and other muscles have to spring into action to compensate.

Using the appropriate amount of weight will help keep you injury-free. The weights used in the Alternating Lateral Raise should not be as heavy as those used in the preceding exercise because it is already more challenging. (Take a look at Chapter 3, where I address how to increase weight safely.)

Getting set

Stand with your feet slightly apart and contract your abs. Holding a light dumbbell in each hand, raise both arms out to the side and up until your arms are even with your shoulders and parallel to the floor. Your palms should be facing down (see Figure 7-3A). Keep your elbows slightly bent and your arms just below shoulder height throughout the entire exercise.

Keep your butt tucked under, abs held tight, and remember not to arch your back.

The exercise

Slowly lower one arm down to your side (see Figure 7-3B) and slowly raise it back up. Then do the same thing with the other arm. Do one or two sets of eight to ten repetitions for each arm. As you progress you can do two or three sets of eight to ten repetitions with increased weight.

During the Alternating Lateral Raise, exhale as your raise the weight up, inhale as you return to start.

Other options

Reduce the weight: If this exercise is too difficult, use less or even no weight.

Sit down: For more of a challenge, do the exercise from a seated position. Once the move is mastered, slightly increase the dumbbell weight.

Bend your elbows: For greater ease, do the exercise with your elbows bent at a 90-degree angle. Although this option is not quite as effective as the original move, it provides a safer alternative for people prone to shoulder injuries.

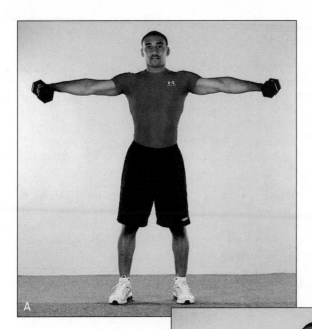

Figure 7-3:
The Alternating Lateral Raise also works the medial deltoid.

Deltoid Press

This exercise is great for your whole shoulder area. It directly targets the front, top, and center deltoids while indirectly hitting the triceps and upper back muscles. Add it to your repertoire of "do anywhere, anytime" shoulder exercises.

Getting set

Sit at the end of a bench or chair with a dumbbell in each hand. If you don't have dumbbells, grab a couple of books or any objects that are similar in size and weight. Your feet should rest comfortably on the floor. Raise your arms to shoulder height with bent elbows. With palms facing out, hold the dumbbells between chin and ear level (see Figure 7-4A).

Keep your back in neutral alignment, which just means that your posture is tall and straight. I explain proper posture in Chapter 1.

The exercise

Press the weights straight up until your arms are almost straight overhead (see Figure 7-4B). Note that there's no need to bang the weights together — that's just a macho thing. Slowly lower the weights back down to the starting position. Do one or two sets of eight to ten repetitions. As you progress, you can move on to doing two or three sets of eight to ten repetitions.

Exhale when you press or lift the weights up. Inhale as you return to start.

If a full-length mirror happens to be nearby, use it! Watch to see if you are doing the correct form I described.

Other options

Use a neutral grip: If you are a beginner, or if you've experienced a shoulder injury, try the exercise with a neutral grip. A neutral grip in this case means that your palms will be facing each other instead of facing out. It's not quite as effective, but it does put less stress on your shoulder joint.

Try a Rotation Press: For more of a challenge, hold the dumbbells with an underhand grip — so that your palms are facing toward you. As you lift, rotate the dumbbells inwards from your shoulders, ending with your palms facing out.

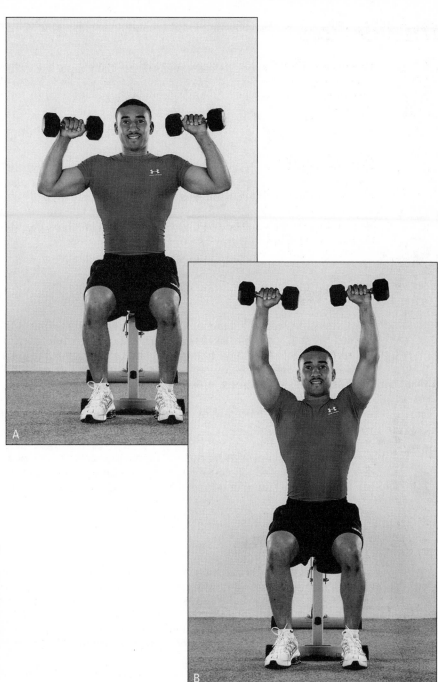

Figure 7-4:
The Deltoid
Press Lift
works the
top and
center of
your
shoulders.

Upright Row

This exercise works your deltoids, your upper back muscles, and, indirectly, your biceps.

Getting set

Stand with your feet shoulder-width apart and your knees slightly bent. Hold a dumbbell in each hand down in front of your legs, with your palms facing your thighs and your arms fully extended (see Figure 7-5A).

Be sure to balance your body weight. Leaning too much on one side or rocking back and forth will throw off your balance.

The exercise

Using slow and controlled movements, raise your upper arms until they are parallel to the floor. Your fists and forearms should be pointing down (see Figure 7-5B). Hold for a few seconds and then slowly return to start. Do one or two sets of eight to ten repetitions. As you progress, you can do two or three sets of eight to ten repetitions with increased weight.

When doing the Upright Row, exhale as you lift the dumbbells and inhale as you return to start.

Avoid using jerky movements, they could mean that you are using weights that are too heavy, which cause an injury. Use only the amount of weight you can handle while still maintaining the described correct form.

Other options

Use a neutral grip: You can make the Upright Row easier by holding the weights with a neutral grip, meaning in this case that your palms are facing each other, and then raising your shoulders up and down as if shrugging.

Try an Alternating Upright Row: For an advanced move, do this exercise one arm at a time.

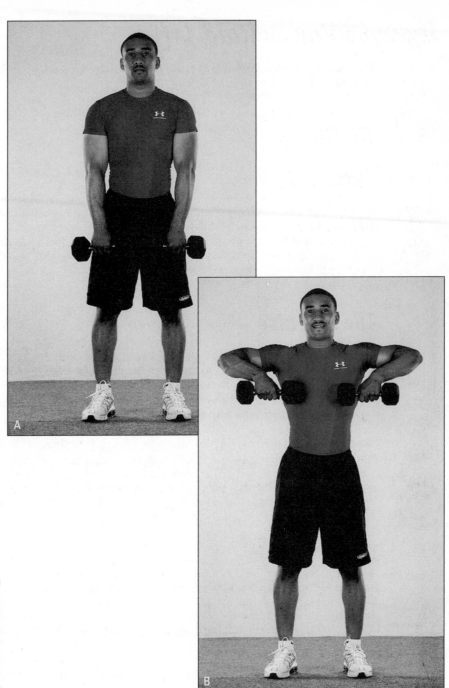

Figure 7-5:
The Upright Row develops your deltoids and upper back.

Seated Rear Deltoid Lift

This exercise works the posterior and medial deltoid muscles and helps strengthen the entire back.

If you have neck problems, you may want to skip this exercise. Try one of the other great shoulder exercises in this chapter.

Getting set

Sit at the end of a bench or chair, with a dumbbell in each hand. Lean forward until your chest is almost parallel to the floor. Try to reach your chest to your legs. Keep your feet flat on the floor and close together. Hold the weights behind your calves with palms facing each other. The weights should almost touch each other (see Figure 7-6A).

The exercise

Extend your arms out to the side and up, with elbows slightly bent as if to form an arc. Raise the weight to shoulder height. Keep your shoulder blades squeezed together. Pause. Return to start (see Figure 7-6B). Do one or two sets of eight to ten repetitions. As you progress, you can do two or three sets of eight to ten repetitions with increased weight.

Exhale when you are exerting force or when you lift the weight up. Inhale as you return to start.

Directing the movement of your shoulders forward keeps the Seated Rear Deltoid Lift movement focused on the rear deltoid rather than on your back.

Other options

Reduce the weight: To simplify the exercise, use less or even no weight.

Stand up: For variety, perform the exercise from a standing position, with your feet hip-width apart. Bend from the hips to form a 45-degree angle with the floor.

Pause longer: To increase the difficulty, hold the pause in the exercise to a slow count of four before returning to start.

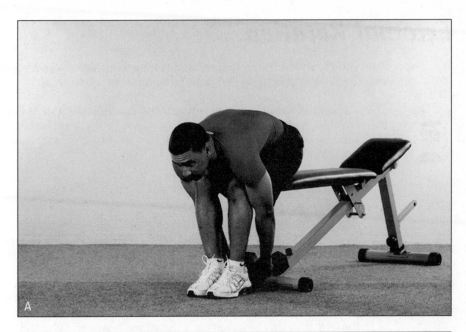

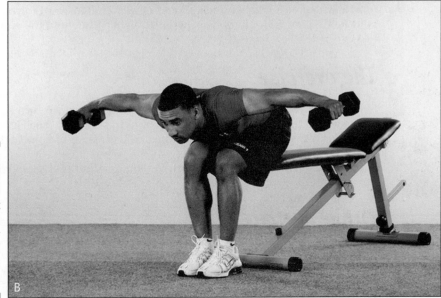

Figure 7-6:
The Seated
Rear Deltoid
Lift
strengthens
your rear
and medial
deltoids and
entire back.

External Rotation

Told you I wouldn't forget that rotator cuff deep in your shoulder joint. This exercise is sure to help you strengthen that injury-prone area.

You will need a tubular resistance band with handles, such as one of those made by Spri. It should be available from any sporting goods store (see Chapter 3 for more). If you can't find this, try the other option, using dumbbells, mentioned after the exercise.

Getting set

Tie one end of the resistance band around a sturdy base such as a pole, a handrail from a staircase, or anything sturdy that is close to waist level. The knot need not be fancy. Simply slip one end of the band through the handle around the base. Stand at a distance equal to the length of the band and pivot your body so that either side is toward the base. Your feet should be hip-width apart. Take the opposite end of the band and hold it with the arm that is farthest away from the base. Keep the elbow bent and close to the body to form a 90-degree angle. Your fist should be centered forward to your body at start (see Figure 7-7A). Keep your wrist straight throughout the entire move.

The exercise

Slowly move your forearm outward to the side and slowly return to start as you maintain the 90-degree angle throughout the exercise (see Figure 7-7B). Do one or two sets of 10 to 15 repetitions on both sides of your body.

Stand tall and straight. Keep your abs in tight and butt tucked under.

Other options

Decrease the resistance: To make the move easier, stand closer to the base of the band. This will decrease the resistance. The further you stand away from the base, the more difficult the move becomes. Always use the correct form that I describe.

Use dumbbells: You can do this move anywhere. For variety, stand with your feet hip-width apart. Holding a dumbbell in each hand, bend your elbows so that your arms form 90-degree angles. Keep the elbows bent and next to your waist for the entire exercise. Your palms should be in front of your body facing the ceiling to start. Keep your shoulder blades squeezed together as you slowly move your arms out to the sides of your body. Return to start. Repeat ten times.

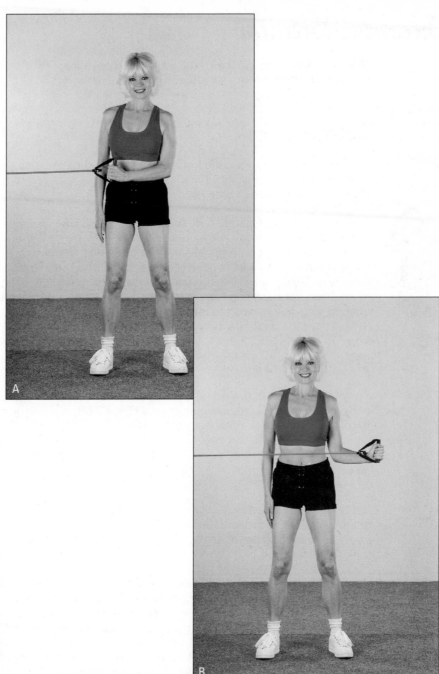

Figure 7-7:
External
Rotation, not
surprisingly,
works your
external
rotators.

Internal Rotation

This exercise is very similar to the preceding one, except that it develops the internal rotator muscles instead of the external ones.

Getting set

Start out the same as External Rotation (see preceding exercise). This time, however, hold the resistance band with the arm that is *closest* to the base with your fist to the side (see Figure 7-8A).

You will need to step a little farther away from the base to provide resistance.

Stand erect as if you were a puppet being pulled by a string from the top of your head. Hold your abs in tight, and butt tucked under. Keep the shoulders relaxed and not raised up toward your ears. The elbows should be bent and close to your body throughout the movement.

The exercise

Slowly move forearm inward until it reaches just beyond the center of your body and then slowly return to start (see Figure 7-8B). Do one or two sets of 10 to 15 repetitions on both sides of the body.

Other options

Decrease the resistance: To make the move easier, stand closer to the base of the band. This will decrease the resistance. The further you stand away from the base the more difficult the move becomes. Always use the correct form that I describe.

Use dumbbells: You can do this move anywhere. For variety, stand with your feet hip-width apart holding a dumbbell in each hand. Bring both arms up and out to the sides at shoulder level, bending your elbows up at a 90-degree angle, so that your palms face forward. Keep your elbows still and pointed straight out from your shoulders as you rotate your arms so that the forearms go down, with the palms facing down, and then bring them slowly back up. Go only as far as is comfortable. Repeat ten times.

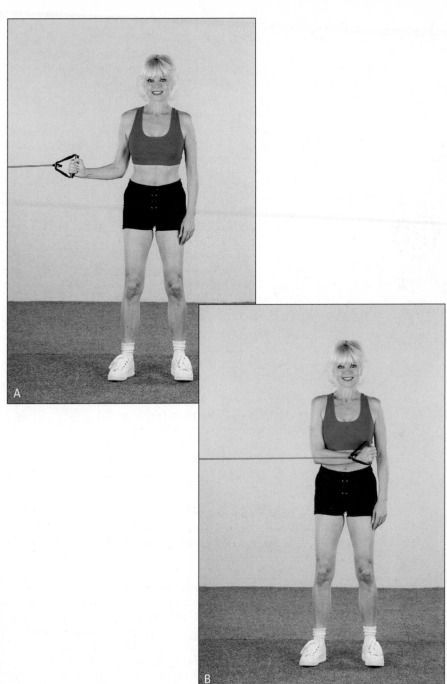

Figure 7-8:
Internal
Rotation
works your
internal
rotators.

Chapter 8

Waving Goodbye to Flabby Arms

• •

In This Chapter

▶ Basic arm anatomy

▶ Why strengthening your arms is beneficial

▶ Toning the arms quickly

▶ Avoiding common arm workout pitfalls

• •

Arm muscles carry a lot of weight in everyday activities. Whether you are lifting a child, reaching for something, or surfing the Internet, arm muscles are being stimulated. Keeping your arm muscles strong not only helps you carry more shopping bags, it also helps you avoid many injuries such as shoulder problems, tennis elbow, or carpal tunnel syndrome of the wrist. *Carpal tunnel syndrome* is an injury caused by movements that are overly repeated, such as too much typing on the computer, overuse of your PlayStation, and excessive knitting.

Buff arms are not too hard on the eyes either. Developing strong arm muscles can also help speed up the results of your chest, shoulder, and back workouts. Those muscles depend on your arms to assist in their respective movements. Take advantage of the extra lift that strong arms can give you for your entire upper body workout. (See Chapters 5, 6, and 7 for more on working out your chest, shoulders, and upper back).

The arm program in this chapter shows you how you can get your arm muscles in shape. After consistently doing these exercises, you can improve your arm strength and muscle tone and show off your arms with confidence at the next barbecue, pool party, or social event. Who knows — you might even choose to make an appearance in a sleeveless shirt or tank top.

Getting to Know Your Arm Muscles

Arming yourself with knowledge of anatomy prepares you for your workout. Whether your arms look like Popeye's or Olive Oyl's, understanding your muscles helps you achieve your personal best shape and strength. As you read about the following arm muscles, compare your own arms with the ones in Figure 8-1. Make a mental note of what you feel as you bend and straighten out these powerful appendages. A mind and body connection really can speed up your results. (Refer to Chapter 2 for a crash course on how to create a mental and physical plan for your arm muscles.)

Following is a breakdown of your arm muscles:

- **Bending with biceps:** The *biceps brachii* muscle, made up of two segments, called the *long head* and the *short head,* covers the front part of your upper arm. Think of a body builder flexing his arms, and you can easily get the pumped-up picture. People commonly call this muscle the *biceps,* and that's the only name you need to remember (see Figure 8-1). The biceps muscle bends your arm at your elbow.

- **Talking about triceps:** You can find the *triceps brachii* directly opposite your biceps. The muscle runs up the rear part of your upper arm and is made up of three sections. Most people simply call it the *triceps* (see Figure 8-1). The triceps muscle makes your arm straighten out at the elbow.

- **Assessing wrist management:** You can find numerous little muscles in your forearm between your elbow and hand. To help you manage these complicated muscle names, so you can ignore any complex mumble jumble; I've grouped them together under a term we all can relate to: *wrist muscles* (see Figure 8-1). The wrist muscles move your wrists in a number of different directions and keep them still when you don't want them to move.

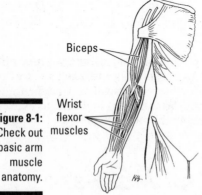
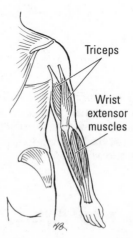

Biceps

Triceps

Wrist extensor muscles

Wrist flexor muscles

Figure 8-1: Check out basic arm muscle anatomy.

Arm Exercise Techniques

It is important to pay attention to proper arm exercise techniques.

Don't forget to start your arm routine with an aerobic warm-up and stretch at the end of your workout. (reach to Chapter 4 for some effective arm stretches).

The only home equipment you need for the arm workouts in this chapter is something to use as a workout bench and a set of inexpensive dumbbells. You can certainly find these at any sporting goods store. Heck, you probably have a step bench or a stool that's strong enough to use as workout bench. Water bottles and canned goods can also make excellent weights in a pinch. (See Chapter 3 for more on this and other equipment.)

Arm exercises are much more effective when you breathe properly. Exhale during the most difficult part of the exercise — during exertion. You should inhale as you prepare to start exerting again.

The following tips help speed your development of strong and contoured arms.

- ✔ **Balance the biceps and triceps:** Make sure to work out both the biceps and triceps muscles. If one is weaker than the other, you are setting yourself up for elbow injuries. Don't fret — I've already put together a balanced, arm exercise menu plan for you. (Use the exercises in this chapter or refer to Chapters 17 and 18 for more great balanced arm workout choices.)

- ✔ **Keep the wrist straight:** Unless you are trying to do a Wrist Curl (see the first exercise in this chapter), where you deliberately bend the wrist up or down, try to maintain a straight wrist during all arm exercises. If you bend your wrist, the resulting strain makes your arm workout less effective and could cause injury.

- ✔ **Avoid rocking:** Whenever I watch people working out at the gym, I'm amazed at how many of them love to rock their bodies back and forth in a million different positions during an arm workout. This inefficient maneuvering works everything *but* the arms. If you find that your body shifts during an arm move, cut back on the weight you're using until you can perform the exercise following the correct form that I describe.

Wrist Curl

Use this move to strengthen the wrist muscles on the inside of your forearm (the palm side). This is perfect for computer users or anyone with injuries caused by repetitive wrist movements.

Getting set

Kneel on the floor facing the long side of the workout bench. Hold a dumbbell in each hand using an underhand grip (palms facing up — find out more about how different grips can affect your arm workout in Chapter 3). Rest your forearms on the bench and let the dumbbells hang over on the opposite side. Let the weights roll down to the tip of your fingers as you open your hands (see Figure 8-2A).

If you have bony knees, try kneeling on a carpet or a towel for more comfort.

The exercise

Curl the dumbbells up toward your forearms as you roll your wrists up to close your hands (see Figure 8-2B). Return to start. Do one or two sets of eight to ten repetitions. As you progress, work up to two or three sets of eight to ten repetitions with increased weight.

Other options

Do it while seated: You can do Wrist Curls anywhere while in a chair. This exercise makes for a perfect break from working at your computer. Just grab your cellphone or any weighted object (don't worry, no airtime minutes will be added on). Lean forward and allow the weight to hang off your knee rather than a bench. Use your other hand to hold your working arm in place. Do the same movement as described in the Wrist Curl. Be sure to do both wrists. This is also an excellent option for people who find the kneeling move too difficult or painful.

Keep your fingers closed: If the Wrist Curl is too difficult, try it without opening your hands. Just curl the wrist up and down without rolling the weight to your fingertips.

Increase the weight: As you become stronger, try doing the move with more weight. But only increase the weight if you can maintain good form and control throughout the entire exercise.

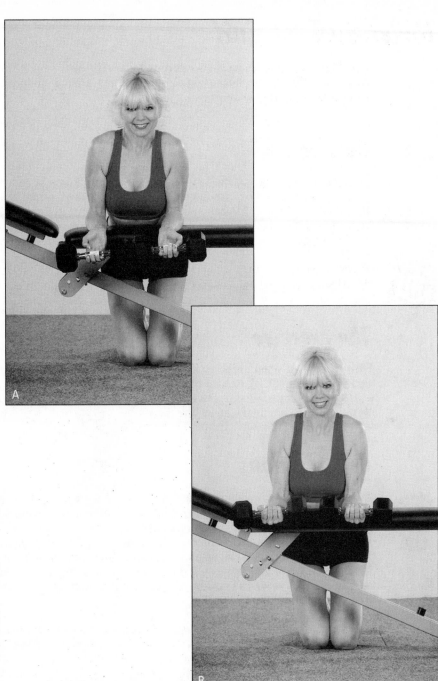

Figure 8-2:
Strengthen
your wrist
muscles
with this
effective
move.

Reverse Wrist Curl

This exercise strengthens the wrist muscles on the outside of your forearm (the same side as your knuckles). Reverse Wrist Curls can help you avoid repetitive wrist muscle injuries.

Getting set

Kneel on the floor facing the long side of the workout bench. Hold a dumbbell in each hand with an overhand grip (palms facing down — find out more about how different grips can affect your arm workout in Chapter 3). Rest your forearms on the bench so that the dumbbells hang over on the opposite side (see Figure 8-3A). Do not open your fingers for this exercise.

The Reverse Wrist Curl usually requires less weight than the Wrist Curl described in the previous exercise.

The exercise

Slowly use your wrist muscles to lift the dumbbells till they are parallel to the floor (see Figure 8-3B). Return to start. Do one or two sets of eight to ten repetitions. As you progress, work up to two or three sets of eight to ten repetitions with increased weight.

Other options

Do it while seated: Take advantage of this timesaving move. In less than two minutes, you can hold on to a can of hairspray or shaving cream and do this exercise, which could protect your wrists from injury. It's the same Reverse Wrist Curl except you perform it while sitting and using one weight, one arm at a time. Lean forward and allow the weight to hang off your knee rather than a bench. Use your other hand to hold your working arm in place. Be sure to do both wrists. This is also an excellent option for people who find it too difficult or painful to kneel.

Shorten the distance: If your wrists are weak, do the same move for a shorter distance.

Increase the weight: As you become stronger, try doing the move with more weight. But only increase the weight if you can maintain good form and control throughout the entire exercise.

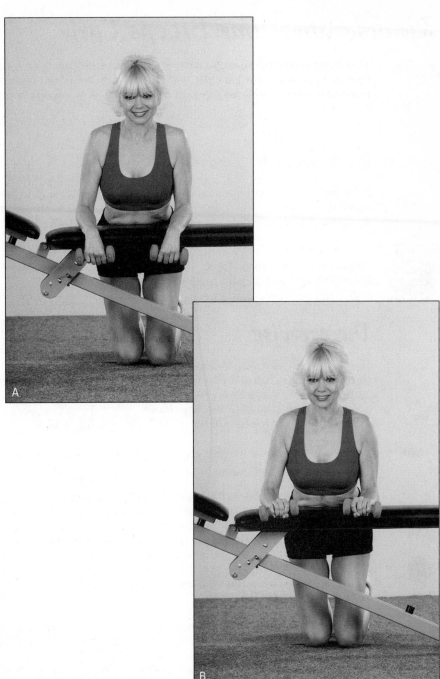

Figure 8-3:
Do the
Reverse
Wrist Curl
while at
your desk.

Seated Same-Time Biceps Curl

This classic exercise shapes and strengthens the biceps muscle and can be done anywhere. Just use a chair instead of a bench. Instead of dumbbells use any handy objects that are equal in weight such as two water bottles or two cans of hairspray.

Getting set

Sit at the end of a workout bench. Hold two dumbbells down at your sides using an underhand grip (palms facing forward — check out Chapter 3 for more gripping information for your arms). See Figure 8-4A.

Sit erect with your back straight and head lifted tall. Do not arch your back. Hold your abdominals in tight. If you find yourself leaning back, you are probably using dumbbells that are too heavy, so lighten up!

The exercise

Slowly curl (lift) the dumbbells up just past your chest and toward your shoulders. At the top of the movement, pause for a second to contract (squeeze) your biceps muscles (see Figure 8-4B). Slowly return to start. Do one or two sets of eight to ten repetitions. As you progress, work up to two or three sets of eight to ten repetitions with increased weight.

Exhale as you curl the weights and work the biceps arm muscles. Inhale as you return to start.

Keep your upper arms next to your sides throughout the entire move. This keeps the concentration on the biceps muscles.

Never rock your body back and forth out of correct form.

Other options

Alternate arms: Try doing the original exercise one arm at a time. Alternating arms for each repetition is easier than exercising both arms at the same time.

Do separate sets on one arm at a time: Doing all the repetitions with one arm before switching to the other one is more difficult than doing both arms at the same time. Never rock your body back and forth out of correct form.

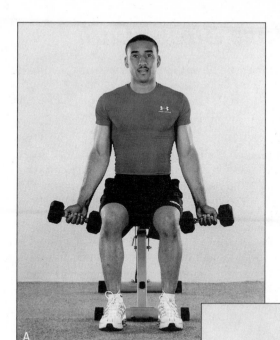

Figure 8-4:
This classic
move
shapes and
strengthens
the biceps.

Angled Same-Time Biceps Curl

This exercise works the entire biceps muscle as well as the forearm.

Getting set

Stand with your feet planted firmly on the ground, hip-width apart. Hold your arms down at your sides with a dumbbell in each hand. Keep your elbows next to your body for the duration of the exercise. Your palms should face outward so that the dumbbells are also outward at an angle from your body (see Figure 8-5A).

Stand tall and erect. Do not lean forward — you could put too much stress on the back. The biceps should do all the work.

The exercise

Slowly lift the dumbbells at the same time until they reach shoulder height. Pause and hold for a second at the top of the move (see Figure 8-5B). Contract or squeeze your biceps muscles and slowly return to start. Do one or two sets of eight to ten repetitions. As you progress, work up to two or three sets of eight to ten repetitions with increased weight.

Exhale as you lift the dumbbells up to your shoulders. Inhale as you return back to start. Do not hold your breath.

Other options

Do it while seated: To simplify the move, try doing it from a seated position. Sitting supports the back and makes it easier to keep your balance.

Alternate arms: Alternating one arm at a time for each repetition is easier than using both arms at the same time.

Do separate sets on one arm at a time: Doing all the repetitions on one arm before switching to the other one is more difficult than doing both arms at the same time.

Keep your wrists straight to avoid injury and to enhance the effect of the move. Straight wrists help strengthen your forearm and wrist muscles.

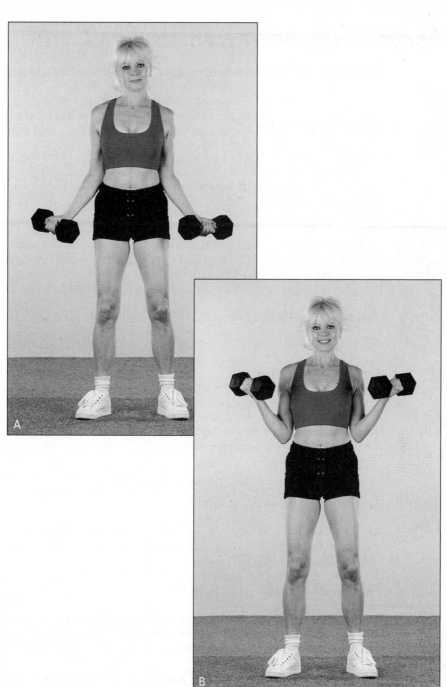

Figure 8-5:
This move
targets the
biceps and
forearm.

Seated Concentration Biceps Curl

The Seated Concentration Biceps Curl is aptly named. It concentrates on the biceps without using the other muscles.

Avoid doing this exercise if you have elbow injuries or experience low back pain. (Review Chapter 1 for more on how health, medical, and safety issues can affect your arm workout.)

Getting set

Sit on a workout bench and hold a dumbbell in your right hand. Your feet should be placed on the floor, slightly wider than hip-width apart. Bend forward from your hips slightly so that your right arm with the weight is hanging straight down and resting against your inner right thigh. The weight should be close to your ankle. Rest your left hand on your left thigh (see Figure 8-6A).

Don't round your back to lean forward. Bend from your hips.

The exercise

Curl the weight up toward your shoulder (see Figure 8-6B). Slowly return to start. Be sure not to bend your wrist or shift your upper torso throughout the move. Do one or two sets of eight to ten repetitions. As you progress, do two or three sets of eight to ten repetitions with increased weight. Alternate arms with each set.

Exhale as you curl the weight up toward your shoulder. Inhale as you return to start.

Other options

Decrease the weight: Simplify the move by using less weight.

Do it standing: To make this move more advanced, try doing it from a standing position. It requires more stability than the seated version. Stand with your feet wider than shoulder-width to help maintain balance.

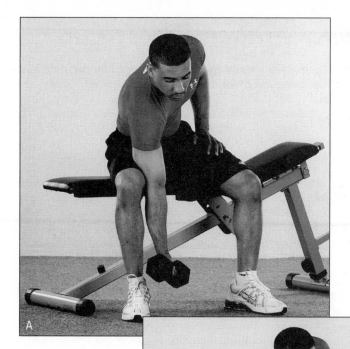

Figure 8-6:
This
exercise
concen-
trates
exclusively
on the
biceps.

Triceps Dip

This is one of the best timesaving exercises ever. You can do it anywhere and experience the benefits of working out your triceps, shoulders, and chest in this one move.

Getting set

With your back to a chair, sofa, or workout bench, firmly place your hands on the surface of the seat. Use your arms to lift your hips off the seat. Straighten out your legs out in front of you with your toes pointing toward the ceiling. Straighten out your arms, but not all the way — keep your elbows slightly bent. Hold your abdominal muscles in tight (see Figure 8-7A).

The exercise

Bend your elbows and slowly lower your body weight till your elbows reach a 90-degree angle or your arms are parallel to the floor. Your lower body should remain in a straight line (see Figure 8-7B). Raise yourself back up to start. If you are new to exercising, start out with one set of five or fewer repetitions. Gradually add on one or two repetitions. Work up to 3 sets of 8 to 12 repetitions.

Do not let your hips do all the moving. Use your elbows for the up and down motion, keeping your wrists straight. The hips and back should be close to the chair, sofa, or bench throughout the movement.

Other options

Make it easier: Bend your knees so that they are at a right angle. It's the same position as if you were sitting in a chair. This is simpler than doing the move with the legs extended.

Make it harder: Rest your feet on another bench that is of equal height to the one you are leaning on.

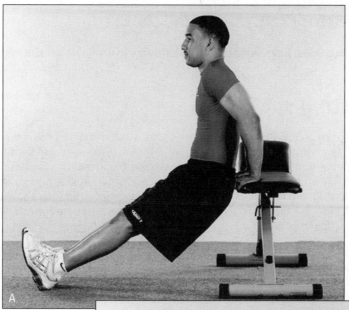

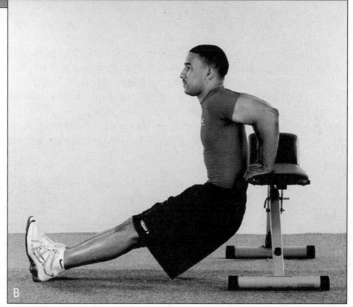

Figure 8-7:
The Triceps
Dip is a
time-crunch
winner.

One-Sided Triceps Kickback

The One-Sided Triceps Kickback is a great way to work out the triceps.

Getting set

Stand next to the left side of a bench with a dumbbell in your left hand. Place your right knee on the bench and bend forward to rest your right hand on the bench for support. Your upper body should be parallel to the floor. Bend the left elbow so that the forearm is perpendicular to the floor (see Figure 8-8A). Be sure to keep the elbow close to your waist. Hold the dumbbell with a neutral grip (palm facing in). (Refer to Chapter 3 for more on how grips affect your arm workout.)

Keep your abs pulled in tight and your back straight (refer to Chapter 1 for more on posture).

The exercise

Slowly raise the dumbbell until your arm is extended straight out behind you (see Figure 8-8B). Don't let your upper arms raise higher or lower than waist level. Pause and hold for a few seconds. Focus on contracting or squeezing your triceps muscle (for more on making a mind-body connection to enhance your arm muscles, review Chapter 2). Slowly return to start. Do one or two sets of eight to ten repetitions one each side. As you progress, work up to two or three sets of eight to ten repetitions with increased weight on each side.

Inhale at the start of the One-Sided Triceps Kickback. Exhale as you lift the dumbbell and inhale when you return to start.

Other options

Twist your palms while lifting: When you lift the weight up behind you, twist your palm so that it faces up. This is a more challenging option.

Two-Sided Triceps Kickback: Begin standing in the same position as the Bent Forward Row (an upper back exercise found in Chapter 6). Keep your feet apart, your lower back slightly arched, and your knees bent. Bend from your hips so that your upper body is almost parallel to the floor. With a dumbbell in each hand, push your forearms straight back. Do not move your upper arms.

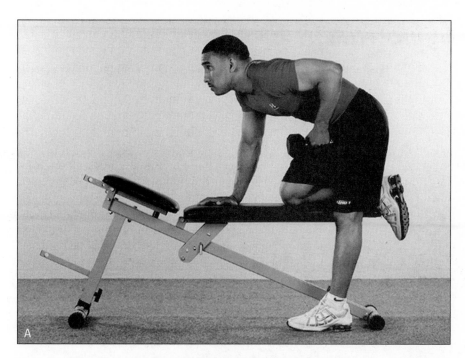

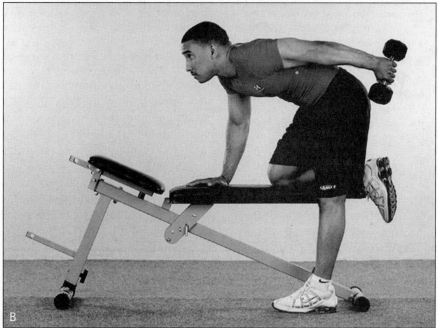

Figure 8-8:
This Kickback works the triceps.

Lying Triceps Extension

It's no lie: The Lying Triceps Extension is a very effective triceps exercise.

Getting set

Lying on your back on a bench, hold two dumbbells above your head with straight arms, your palms facing in. Keep your feet flat on the floor, hip-width apart (see Figure 8-9A).

For more comfort, feel free to place your feet on top of the bench.

The exercise

Keep your shoulders stable as you slowly bend your elbows to lower the weight to the side of your head (see Figure 8-9B). Return to start. Do one or two sets or eight to ten repetitions. As you progress, do two or three sets of eight to ten repetitions with increased weight.

Don't let your arms go lower than just below 90 degrees. Doing so could harm the elbow joint. And be careful not to arch your back.

Inhale at the start of the Lying Triceps Extension. Exhale as you lift the weights up toward the ceiling.

Other options

Do it with one arm: It's easier if you do the Lying Triceps with one arm and one weight at a time.

Alternate arms: Keep one weight in the up position while the other one does the exercise, and then keep alternating positions. This is a more difficult option.

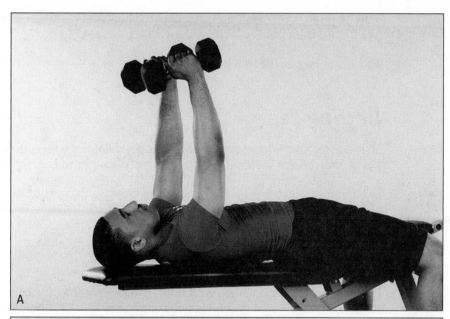

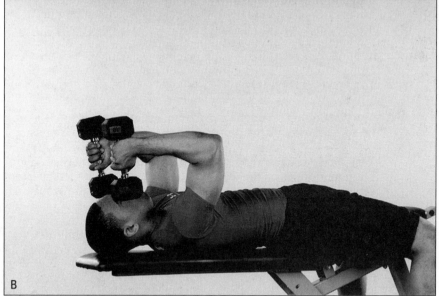

Figure 8-9:
The Lying
Triceps
Extension
is difficult
but very
effective.

Over-the-Head Triceps Extension

This move targets the triceps muscle.

Getting set

Sit at the end of a workout bench and hold one dumbbell with both hands over your head. Be sure to keep the elbows close to your head (see Figure 8-10A).

Hold your stomach in and sit tall and straight. Visualize a string holding you up from the top of your head. Do not arch your back.

The exercise

Keeping your elbows close to your head, slowly lower the dumbbell back behind your head until your forearms are parallel to the floor (see Figure 8-10B). Slowly return to start.

Exhale as you lift the weight up over your head. Inhale as you return to start.

Other options

Try it standing: Doing the move from a standing position is more advanced. Be sure to maintain the proper posture I explain in the exercise.

Vary the count: For variety, try the move using a variety of counts. For example, count to two on the way back and count up to four as you return to start, or vice versa.

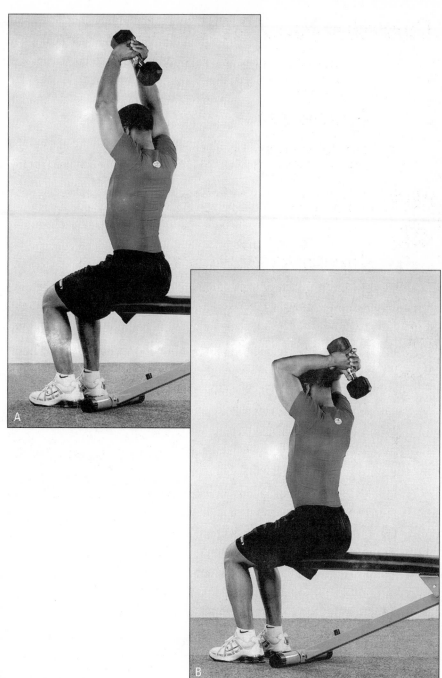

Figure 8-10:
Over-the-
Head is an
effective
triceps
move.

Part III
Lower-Body Workouts

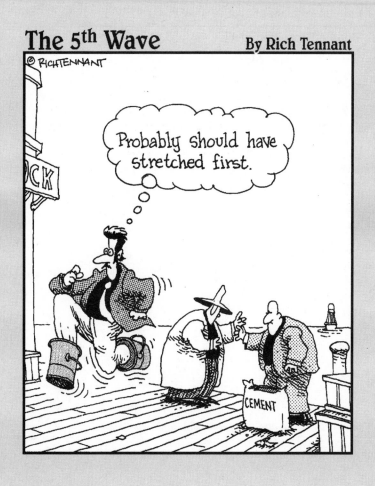

The 5th Wave   By Rich Tennant

Probably should have stretched first.

CEMENT

In this part . . .

Here you'll discover the joy of having sculpted buns, legs, and calves. I've selected exercises that deliver winning muscle definition for your lower body. I also give you basic anatomy information so you can focus on and visualize the muscles you're working on. And I provide you with tips on technique to contribute to fast results while avoiding injury.

Chapter 9

Lightening Up Thunderous Thighs

· ·

In This Chapter

▶ Checking out basic thigh anatomy

▶ Discovering techniques and tips for terrific thighs

▶ Performing thigh exercises

· ·

The thighs are an amazing construction of muscle groups that work together as a whole rather than a microcosm of individual parts. You can, however, target your specific problem areas with exercises that emphasize or isolate the particular thigh muscle you want to work on. In this chapter, I show you fast and effective exercises that tone the inner and outer thighs. (To target the muscles of the front and back of your thighs as well as your buns, check out Chapters 10 and 11.)

Making your inner and outer thighs the right size has both physical and practical benefits. Bringing your legs together to stand tall so that you can impress a date in the theater line, crossing one leg over the other to play soccer, or dancing the two-step requires the inner thigh muscles. Lifting your leg out to the side to go skating, dancing, or to trip a friend uses the outer thigh muscles. Strengthening the inner and outer thigh muscles helps to prevent hip injuries — a prevalent problem among seniors. In fact, just about any lower body leg activity (running, walking, jumping, and so on) is improved with strong inner and outer thighs.

Both men and women look ten times better when the inner and outer thighs are toned up. There are men who pump their upper body in excess only to be left standing on two underdeveloped limbs making them look totally out of balance. Some women have an unfounded fear of developing bulky thighs and instead opt for the not so popular saddlebag spread, which is a direct result from sitting too much. Others think that the thighs will just magically disappear when the truth is you cannot spot reduce. Thankfully, there are many areas on your thighs that you can tone up and improve their visual appeal immensely. Results can vary depending on your genetic body type and muscle fiber variations (Chapter 2 explains how understanding your body type and muscle fiber makeup can help you set realistic goals). Choose to reach your personal best inner and outer thigh proportions.

Getting to Know Your Thighs

Understanding the basic anatomy of your thighs can aid in visualizing your specific goals (Chapter 2 has more on the power of positive visualization). Following is a simple description of the inner and outer thigh muscles used in this chapter. Balance your thigh workout with exercises for the quadriceps, hamstrings, buns, and calves (see Chapters 10 to 12).

Figure 9-1 highlights the muscles of the inner and outer thighs.

✔ **Adding up the adductors:** Several muscles stretch from the inside of your hips to many places along your inner thigh. It serves no purpose to name all of them. Most experts can't. They are referred to as the *adductors.* To avoid confusion, it's easier to simply call them your inner thighs. You use them to squeeze your legs onto a bucking bronco as you hold on for your dear life. Anytime you bring those legs together, it's the inner thighs that are working (see Figure 9-1).

✔ **Admiring the abductors:** Along the side of your hips is a group of muscles called the *abductors.* The abductor muscles are made up of two meaty muscles called the *gluteus medius* and the *gluteus minimus.* Don't get hung up on this technical jargon. Everybody calls them the outer thighs — you can, too. They are responsible for moving your legs away from your body, such as when you are playing hockey or doing side kicks (see Figure 9-1).

Adductors

Abductors

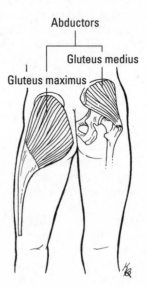

Gluteus medius

Gluteus maximus

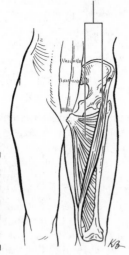

Figure 9-1:
Visualize
your own
thigh
muscles.

Thigh Exercise Techniques

Keep the following in mind if you want to achieve fabulous thighs in little time:

- ✔ **Warm-up and stretch:** Start off your thighs workout with an aerobic warm-up. Be sure to stretch after your routine. (Find specific stretching moves for your thighs in Chapter 4.)

- ✔ **Breathe correctly:** Exhale during the exertion part of an exercise or when the move is most difficult. If you get confused, just keep breathing. Never hold your breath.

- ✔ **Work all your leg muscles:** When you are in a time crunch, it's only natural to focus your workout attention on a problem area such as the inner and outer thighs while excluding other parts of your legs or buns. This can, however, slow down your results because the strength of your leg muscles will be out of balance, and this imbalance makes you more prone to injury. (It is best to include all of the leg and butt muscle exercises in your thigh workout. They can be found in Chapters 10 to 12. For your convenience, there's also a complete leg workout that includes the thighs in Chapters 17 and 18.)

- ✔ **Work large muscle groups:** When you are short on time, try doing exercises that focus on large muscle groups to get a more balanced workout. For example, in a pinch try doing lunges as described in Chapter 10. Not only do they work the thighs but they tone the quads, hamstrings, butt and calves. That single move is more effective than going to the gym, doing a few leg lifts and running out.

- ✔ **Focus on quality not quantity:** For some reason, thigh exercises have the reputation of requiring numerous repetitions in order to be effective. Unfortunately, in an effort to do way too many thigh moves, you can lose the correct form, which sets you up for injury. If you can't consistently do the proper technique that I describe throughout all of the repetitions — stop!

- ✔ **Avoid locking your knees:** Don't lock your knees when doing thigh exercises. Keep them somewhat loose to avoid injury.

- ✔ **Holds your abs in tight:** Hold your abs in tight when you do thigh exercises. A strong core (abs and lower back) enhances the effectiveness of your thigh workout by stabilizing your body so that you can perform a more balanced move. (See Chapters 13 to 16 for information on building a strong core.)

Inner Thigh Leg Lift

Strengthen and sculpt your inner thighs with this exercise.

Getting set

Lie on the floor so that your weight is on your left side. Place your left elbow on the floor, keeping it lined up directly under your shoulder. Gently place the fingertips of your right hand on the ground in front of you — strictly for balance and support. Your right knee should be bent up and facing the ceiling while your right foot is planted on the floor behind the thigh of your left leg (see Figure 9-2A).

The exercise

Using slow and controlled movements, lift your lower leg up until you feel the contraction (squeeze) of your left inner thigh. Hold for a few seconds (see Figure 9-2B). Slowly return to start. Do five to ten repetitions. As you progress, work up to 10 to 20 repetitions. Repeat the exercise on the opposite side.

Hold your abdominals in tight for stability. Keep the leg that you are lifting straight, but do not lock the knees. Do not slouch back on your butt — remain balanced on your hip. Keep the foot that you are lifting flexed and parallel to the floor.

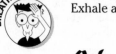

Exhale as you lift your lower leg up. Inhale as you lower it back to the floor.

Other options

Ask a friend: Add resistance to this move by having a friend press down on the calf of your straight leg as you contract your inner thigh to lift your lower leg.

Use an ankle weight: Add resistance with an ankle weight. Pick one up at any sporting goods store (see Chapter 3 for more on equipment).

Use your hand: Use your own hand for resistance. Rather than gently pressing your fingertips into the floor for balance, press your hand into your working thigh for added resistance.

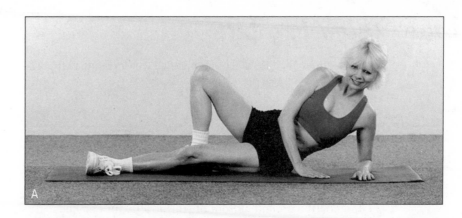

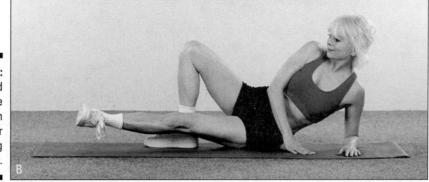

Figure 9-2:
Tone and
sculpt those
thighs with
the Inner
Thigh Leg
Lift.

Outer Thigh Leg Lift

The Outer Thigh Leg Lift is a great exercise that does just what the name implies — works on the outer thigh muscles.

Getting set

Lie on the floor on your left side. Lift your left shoulder straight up so that your elbow is placed directly under it. Bend your lower left knee so that the sole of your left foot is facing behind you. Gently place the fingertips of your right hand on the ground in front of you, strictly for balance and support (see Figure 9-3A).

The exercise

Using slow and controlled movements, raise your upper right leg not more than a few feet off the floor. You should feel the contraction or squeeze of your outer thigh as you lift your leg up (Figure 9-3B). Hold for a few seconds. Slowly return to start. Do five to ten repetitions. As you progress, work up to 10 to 20 repetitions. Repeat the exercise on the opposite leg.

Hold your abdominals in tight for stability throughout the entire move. Keep the leg that you are lifting straight, but do not lock your knee. Resist the temptation to slouch back on your butt. Your posture should be such that you are balanced on the side of your body. Keep the foot that you are working flexed and parallel to the floor.

Exhale as you lift your leg up. Inhale as you lower it to the floor.

Other options

Ask a friend: Have a friend press down on the calf of your straight leg for resistance as you contract the outer thigh of your upper leg to lift it up.

Use an ankle weight: Wrap an ankle weight around your straight leg to add resistance to the movement. These are available at sporting goods stores (see Chapter 3 for more on equipment).

Press your hand: Press your own hand against your leg. Instead of gently pressing your fingertips into the floor for balance, use your hand for resistance against your working thigh.

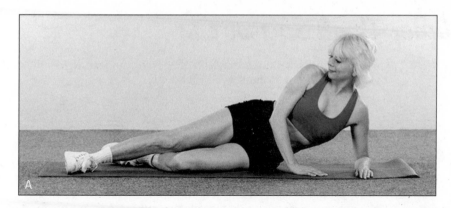

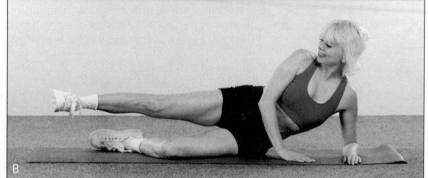

Figure 9-3:
Focus on
the outer
thigh
contraction.

Inner Thigh Scissor Cut

Cut to the chase with this Inner Thigh Scissor Cut that works the adductors, the muscles on the inside of your leg.

Getting set

Lie on your back so that your legs and feet are pointed straight up toward the ceiling. Your arms should be out to the side (see Figure 9-4A).

To avoid any pressure on your back, pay attention to the position of your spine. Do not arch your back, nor for that matter keep it unnaturally flat. Allow for at the most an inch and a half between the floor and your back. (See Chapter 1 where the importance of proper posture is discussed.)

The exercise

Maintaining good posture, open your legs up and out to the side as wide as possible without toppling over or falling down or out of form. Keep your toes pointed as you stretch your inner thighs out at the side (see Figure 9-4B). Now bring your legs together and do two short scissor cuts. First, the left leg should cross over the right at the knees, and then the right leg should quickly cross over the left at the knees (see Figure 9-4C). Return to the wide open leg position. Repeat this pattern five to ten times. As you progress, work up to 10 to 20 repetitions.

To enhance this move, visualize that your legs are being pulled up from your hips and out to the side. When you prepare to bring your legs together to do the scissor-cut cross pattern, keep imagining a force pulling your legs wide apart. This will help you to create more resistance with your inner thigh muscles. This mind over body technique works in a snap.

Other options

Give it extra stretch: You can add an extra stretch to this exercise by placing your hands on your inner thigh and pressing your thighs further out to the side. The resistance from your own body weight helps to increase the stretch.

Use ankle weights: Add resistance to this move with ankle weights. You can pick them up at any sporting goods store. (See Chapter 3 for more on equipment.)

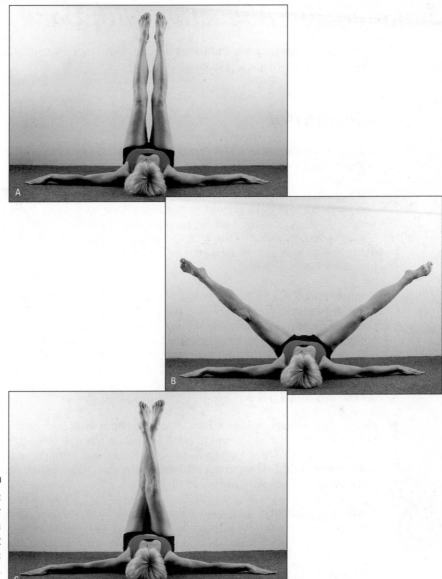

Figure 9-4:
Hold your abdominals in tight during this move.

Standing Hip Abduction with Band

This exercise strengthens and tones the hip abductors, the outer thigh muscles that pull your leg away from your body.

Getting set

For this exercise you need an exercise band that is between 1[bf]1/2 to 2 feet circular. Bands can be found at any sporting goods store (see Chapter 3).

Start by slipping your feet within the circle of the exercise band. Secure the band around your ankles. Holding your hands on your waist, balance your weight on one foot while keeping the band taut (see Figure 9-5A).Many people find it necessary to hold onto a chair when completing this move. That is perfectly fine as long as it is used strictly for balance. See the other options that follow for more details.

Because balance is of the utmost importance to successfully complete this move, it is best to start out the exercise with proper posture and maintain it throughout. Stand tall, stretching from your head to your toes, as if you are being pulled by a string. (See Chapter 1 for posture tips.)

The exercise

Slowly lift and stretch your raised leg out to the side as high as is comfortable. Remain standing tall and upright as you do a series of small side kicks (see Figure 9-5B). Do not try to raise your leg beyond a couple of feet. Hold your abs in tight. Do five to ten repetitions on each side. As you progress, work up to 10 to 20 repetitions.

Achieve the stability you need for this exercise by developing a strong core (abs and lower back). (See Chapters 13 through 16 for core strength moves.)

Other options

Hold on for support: If you find it hard to balance on one leg, hold onto a cane or a broomstick placed directly in front of you or a fixed object such as the wall or a table at your side. Use that object only for balance; keep your spine upright and don't lean over from your waist into the object.

Add ankle weights: You can increase the difficulty of this move by wearing ankle weights at the same time you are wearing the exercise band.

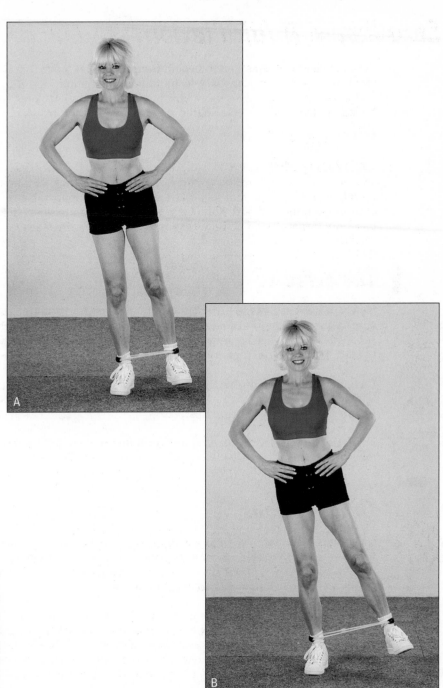

Figure 9-5:
Work the
outer thighs
with this
exercise.

Legs Apart Thigh Flexion

Both men and women stand to benefit from this ballet move that works the inner thighs as well as the quadriceps, glutes, and hamstrings. (Check out Chapters 10 through 12 for more lower body exercises.) Athletes such as hockey and soccer players use this move as part of their training.

Getting set

Start by standing with your legs apart as wide as is comfortable so that your toes are pointing outward. Keep your back straight, shoulders back, and chest out. Arms should be down at your sides (see Figure 9-6A).

The exercise

Slowly flex your thighs to lower them until they are horizontal to the floor. Be sure to keep the knees in a straight line with the toes as you lower the body to avoid knee injury (see Figure 9-6B). Contract your buttocks to help you return to start. Do five to ten repetitions. As you progress, work up to 20 repetitions.

Do not bend forward during this move. Hold your abs in tight for stability. Keep your spine tall and straight for the duration of the exercise. (See Chapter 1 for several posture tips.)

Inhale as you lower your body. Exhale as you exert yourself back to an upright position.

Other options

Use a staff: Rest a staff such as a cane or a broomstick on your shoulder, which can help you keep your back straight. It also works to hold the staff in front of you over your thighs. As you do the exercise, slide it down past your thighs and calves. Remember to maintain proper posture.

Hold the contraction: Make the move more advanced by holding the contraction in the down position for a count of two before returning to start.

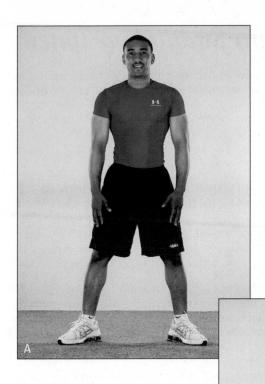

Figure 9-6:
Flexing the thighs helps to sculpt the inside of your legs.

Anytime Standing Saddlebag Toner

Tone up those outer thighs anywhere with the Anytime Standing Saddlebag Toner. Do this while preparing dinner, faxing a document, or while waiting for the laundry to finish.

Getting set

Start by standing tall. Hold your stomach in tight and buttocks tucked under. Your feet should be planted on the floor shoulder-width apart (see Figure 9-7A).

The exercise

Slowly lift and raise one leg out to the side a few feet (see Figure 9-7B). Return to start. Do five to ten repetitions on each side. As you progress or if time permits do 10 to 20 repetitions on each side. Do this move over and over again throughout the day for fast, effective toned-up results. No more excuses!

Exhale as you lift your leg up and inhale as you bring it back down.

Other options

Hold the contraction: Holding the contraction of your outer thigh muscles with your leg in a raised position will increase the difficulty of the Anytime Standing Saddlebag Toner.

Try it on ice skates: Doing this exercise while wearing ice skates, balancing a book on your head, and reciting the *Gettysburg Address* will increase the difficulty of this move — okay, perhaps that's too much!

Make it an inner thigh move: Turn this anytime-anywhere move into an inner thigh exercise. Rather than kicking your leg out to the side, cross one leg over the other as you squeeze your inner thigh muscles. Return to start. Maintain good posture throughout all of the repetitions. Be sure to do both legs.

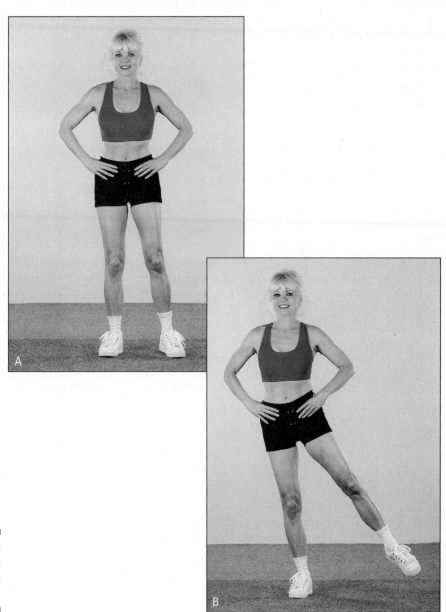

Figure 9-7:
Tone-up
your thighs
anywhere.

Chapter 10

Getting a Leg Up: Hamstrings and Quadriceps

In This Chapter

▶ Understanding hamstrings and quadriceps muscles

▶ Getting tips on exercise techniques

▶ Finding exercises for the hamstrings and quadriceps

Strong hamstrings and quadriceps reap many benefits, with injury prevention at the top of the list. But also, hamstrings and quadriceps exercises provide a fast-fitness return on the effort of your aerobic workout. It has been proven that strong legs can do wonders to increase your stamina and pick up your pace in any number of cardiovascular activities, such as running, jumping, and kickboxing. It also stands to reason that the extra edge derived from the strengthening moves in this chapter provide a calorie-cutting advantage: You get the added benefit of burning calories faster. Last, but not least, strong, toned-up legs simply look fabulous on both men and women. Strengthening and sculpting them provide a balanced physique that is visually appealing in both genders.

So lessen your chance for common joint injuries, improve the effectiveness of your aerobic workout, and make your legs look good just by strengthening hamstrings and quadriceps with the top-notch exercises in this chapter.

Getting to Know Your Hamstrings and Quadriceps

Taking the time to understand the anatomy of your hamstrings and quadriceps can help you achieve faster results. Visualizing the way these muscles move helps you target the specific leg muscle groups you want to work on. Following is a brief discussion about the hamstrings and quadriceps muscles developed by the exercises in this chapter. Remember to balance your lower body leg workout with moves for your inner and outer thighs, buns, and calves.

✔ **Hailing your hamstrings:** On the back of each leg is a group of muscles called the hamstrings. To sound hip to the lingo, call them what those of us in the fitness industry do: the *hams.* To impress former classmates at your next class reunion, call them by their scientific names:

- The **biceps femoris** (outer rear thigh)
- The **semitendinosus** (inner rear thigh)
- The **semimembranosus** (inner rear thigh)

The hamstrings are responsible for any flexion of the knees. That just means that when you bring your heel up to your butt, you are using the hamstrings (and also when sprinting, pulling your legs up the steps, and so on) to get great gams — work the hams! (See Figure 10-1.)

✔ **Qualifying your quadriceps:** This large group of muscles is technically called the *quadriceps femoris* (see Figure 10-1). Most people simply call them the *quads.* The quads are made up of four muscles. If you are studying to become a contestant on a quiz show, the following names might be helpful. Otherwise, *quads* will do. Here are the quads:

- The **vastus lateralis** (on the outside)
- The **vastus medialis** (on the inside)
- The **vastus intermedius** (between the lateralis and the medialis)
- The **rectus femoris** (above the other three quads)

Lifting your leg up to kick, press, or extend from a bent position involves the quadriceps. Having strong quadriceps can literally give you a leg up in life.

Figure 10-1:
It's helpful to remember where your hams and quads are.

Quadriceps

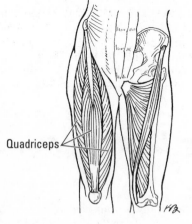
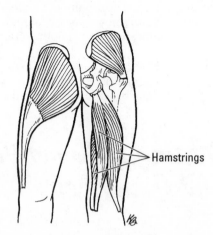

Hamstrings

Hamstrings and Quadriceps Exercise Techniques

Walking through life is a lot easier if you have been practicing good hamstrings and quadriceps techniques. To successfully achieve strong, sculpted hamstrings and quadriceps, follow this advice:

- ✔ **Warm-up and stretch:** Always start your hamstrings and quadriceps workout with an aerobic warm-up. Include stretching after your exercise session. (See Chapter 4 for lower body stretches.)

- ✔ **Remember to exhale:** Exhale during the exertion or most challenging part of a hamstrings and quadriceps exercise. This can sometimes be difficult to differentiate since leg moves involve a mixture of pushing and pulling movements (as in squats, lunges, and curls). Rather than get frustrated, just keep breathing. Never hold your breath.

- ✔ **Balance your leg muscles:** Working your hamstrings and quadriceps may be your primary goal, but including inner and outer thighs, calves, and butt exercises can help you avoid muscle imbalance. Muscle imbalance slows down the results of all your effort. More importantly, it makes you more prone to injury. (Include all the butt and leg muscles in your hams and quads workout — see Chapters 9, 11, and 12. Prepackaged complete leg workouts are in Chapters 17 and 18.)

- ✔ **Keep knees and toes lined up:** When doing leg exercises that require you to lunge or squat, never extend your knees beyond your toes. It is safest to keep them lined up directly on top of each other to avoid joint injury. If you feel pain, stop!

- ✔ **Do not arch your back:** Whether you are squatting, lunging, pressing, or curling (leg exercises), do not arch your back. Keep your vertebrae in neutral alignment, meaning your spine is elongated to follow its natural curve. (See Chapter 1 for proper posture guidelines.)

Lunge

Take the lunge with this fast, effective, anytime-anywhere move. Not only does it do wonders for your quadriceps and hamstrings, but it tones the thighs, butt, and calves.

Getting set

Stand with your feet hip-width apart. Rest your hands on your hips. Hold your abs in tight with your butt tucked under (see Figure 10-2A).

Maintain proper posture for the entire exercise. Elongate the spine from head to toe. (See Chapter 1 for more posture tips.)

The exercise

With your left foot planted on the floor, lift your right leg up so that your toes are pointed forward. Bend both knees as you lunge between two and three feet to the front, lifting your back heel up slightly. The front leg should be parallel to the floor while the back leg is perpendicular. Do not let your right knee move beyond your toes (see Figure 10-2B). Return to start. Do five to ten repetitions. As you progress, work up to 10 to 20 repetitions. Repeat on the other side.

Maintain balance by looking toward the front. Don't lean too far forward or you will topple over. Remember to keep your spine straight.

Other options

Work the inner thigh: To effectively work the inner thigh, perform the lunge to the side at a 45- to 90-degree angle.

Stay in one spot: Simplify the lunge by not returning to the original start position. Lift your body and bend your knees up and down from the forward position.

Move backward: Do the move backwards. This concentrates on the hamstrings.

Use weights: With a weight in each hand, hold your arms down at your side. This increases the difficulty of the move.

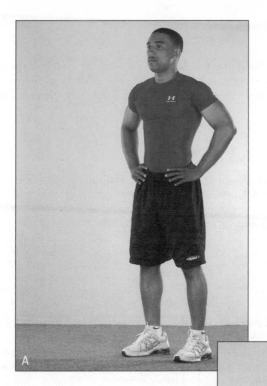

Figure 10-2:
Take the
lunge
forward.

Resistance Band Squat

This exercise targets mainly the quadriceps, hamstrings, and butt muscles. You will need a tubular resistance band such as one of those made by Spri (available at any sporting goods store — see Chapter 3 for more on equipment).

Getting set

Stand with your feet hip-width apart on top of a tubular resistance band. Hold an end of the band in each hand. Bring your fists together over your chest so that the band rests on your upper arms behind your elbows. Bring your elbows out to the side like chicken wings (see Figure 10-3A). Stand tall and hold your abdominals in tight.

The exercise

Slowly bend your knees to bring your body down as if you were going to sit on a chair. Do not lean more than slightly forward or angle your thighs past the point of being parallel to the floor (see Figure 10-3B). Slowly contract (squeeze) your butt and legs as you push or put pressure on your heels to return to start. Do five to ten repetitions. As you progress, work up to 10 to 20 repetitions.

Do not press your knees beyond your toes during the exercise or lock them at the start.

If you are experiencing any pain such as in the lower back or knee — stop! Consult with your physician. It might be best to try the easier choice from the other options provided.

Other options

Use your body weight: If the exercise is too difficult or uncomfortable for you, try it with no band. As you bring your body down to a sitting position, extend your arms out in front of you for balance. Make it even easier by holding onto an object such as the back of a tall chair in front of you.

Use weights: For variety, do the same move with hand-held weights.

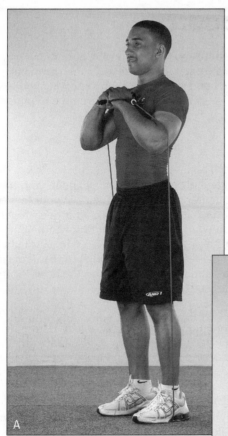

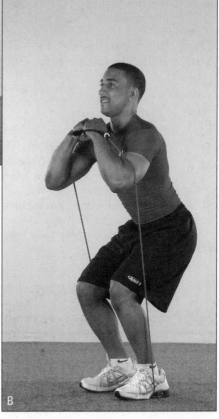

Figure 10-3:
Never bring
your knees
over your
toes.

Great Legs Band Stretch

This is one of those moves that I can't help but rave about. In a minimal amount of time, it hits multiple parts: quadriceps, hamstrings, butt, and inner thighs. Grab your resistance band (available at any sporting goods store from manufacturers such as Spri — see Chapter 3 for more on equipment).

Getting set

Lie on your back. Holding each end of the resistance band in your hands, place the balls of your feet on the center of the band. Turn out your legs by rotating your hips open. Point your toes out to the side with your heels together. Bend and lift your knees up and outward (froglike), shoulder-width apart, directly over and even with your hips. Keep the toes and knees in a straight line to avoid knee joint injury. Your calves should be parallel to the floor, and your feet flexed. Keep your elbows and upper arms flat on the floor for the entire exercise as you hold onto the ends of the band (see Figure 10-4A).

Stabilize this move by slightly tilting the pelvis, squeezing your abdominals, and maintaining contact with your back on the floor.

The exercise

Slowly press your legs straight out while your heels are kept together. Try to keep your legs as low to the floor as possible (see Figure 10-4B). Return to start. Do five to ten repetitions. As you progress, work up to 10 to 20 repetitions.

Do not arch your back or lock your knees and never lift the shoulder or neck.

Exhale as you press your legs out. Inhale when you return to start.

Other options

Reach your arms over your head: Advance this move by doing it with your arms over your head. Be extra careful not to arch your back.

Lighten the resistance: If this move is too difficult, check the resistance of your band. You may be using one that is too heavy for you. Also try to loosen the end of your band. Tightening the band to shorten it increases the resistance, but loosening the band to lengthen it decreases the resistance.

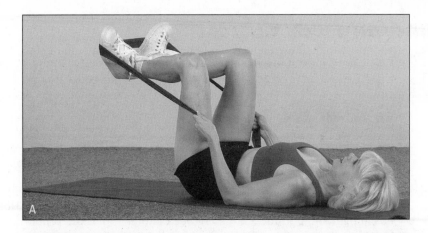

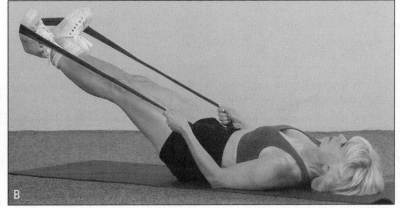

Figure 10-4:
Keep your upper arms stable during this move.

Standing Heel Curl

This classic move does wonders for the backs of your legs, or hamstrings.

Getting set

Stand with your weight on one leg with that knee slightly bent. The opposite leg should be extended out straight behind you. Place your hands on your hips (see Figure 10-5A).

Stand tall so that your head, back, and supporting leg are lined up. Hold the abs in tight and butt tucked under. (See Chapter 1 for more proper posture tips.)

The exercise

Slowly bend the knee of the extended leg and lift the heel of your foot up toward your butt (see Figure 10-5B). Return to start. Do five to ten repetitions. As you progress, work up to 10 to 20 repetitions. Do the move on the opposite leg.

To help maintain balance, be sure to squeeze your hamstrings and butt as you contract your leg to lift your foot.

Exhale as you lift your leg up. Inhale as you return to start.

Other options

Hold for balance: To simplify this exercise, hold onto a sofa or chair for balance.

Use ankle weights: Up the level of difficulty by using ankle weights.

Adjust the count: For variety, lift your leg up for a slow count of four and then down for a slow count of four.

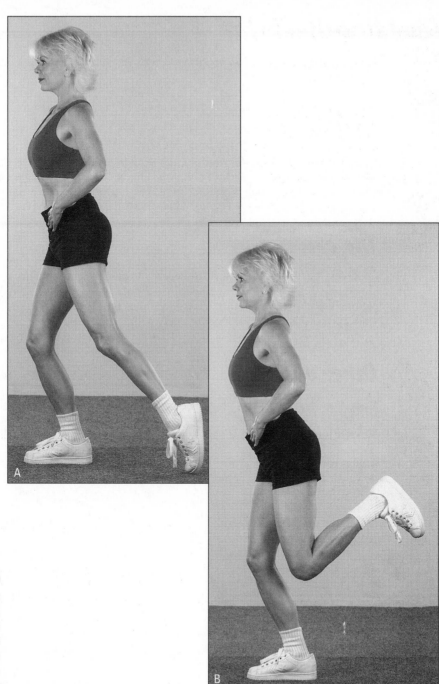

Figure 10-5:
This curl strengthens and tones the hamstrings.

Hamstrings Curl

The Hamstrings Curl tones and strengthens the back of the legs — the hamstrings.

Getting set

Kneel on all fours. Lean forward so that your weight is supported on your elbows and your head is resting on your hands. Your butt is higher than your shoulders, but your pelvis should be tucked under (see Figure 10-6A).

The exercise

Contract your hamstrings and squeeze your butt to bend and lift your right knee up with the heel curling toward your butt. Keep the foot flexed (see Figure 10-6B). Return to start. Do five to ten repetitions. As you progress, work up to 10 to 20 repetitions. Repeat on the opposite leg.

Other options

Make it easier: Lie flat on your stomach to make this move easier.

Make it harder: This move can be more challenging if you add ankle weights.

Adjust the count: For variety, lift the leg up for a slow count of three and down for a faster count of one.

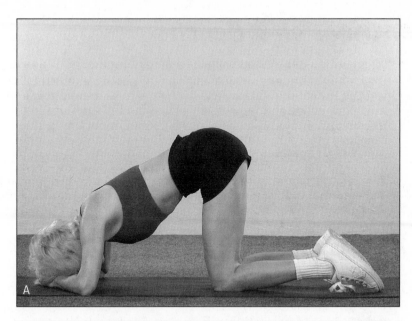

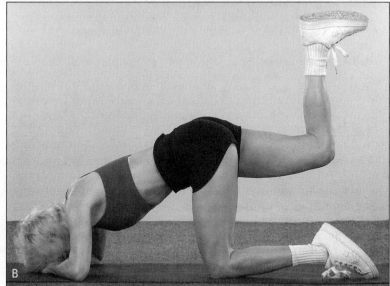

Figure 10-6:
Squeeze
your butt
and
hamstrings
as you curl.

Hamstrings on a Bench

This exercise sculpts your hamstrings and strengthens them at the same time. You will need a home workout bench or any raised platform that is strong enough to hold you and long enough for you to lie on from your knees up.

Getting set

Lie on a bench on your stomach so that your head is up and your weight is supported on your forearms. Your knees should be hanging off the bench with legs extended straight out behind you. Keep the feet flexed (see Figure 10-7A).

Do not arch your back. Hold your abs in tight and butt tucked under.

The exercise

Contract your butt and hamstrings to bring both legs up at the same time toward your rear end (see Figure 10-7B). Return to start. Do five to ten repetitions. As you progress, work up to 10 to 20 repetitions.

Remember to exhale during the most difficult part of this move or when you lift your legs up. Inhale as you return to start.

Other options

Use the floor: To make this move easier, perform it on the floor.

Use weights: Increase the level of difficulty by adding ankle weights or holding a dumbbell between your feet.

Hold the contraction: Make the move more effective by holding the contraction of your hamstrings for a few seconds when your legs are in the up position.

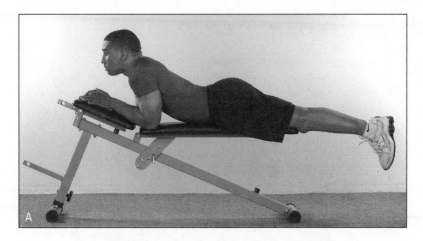

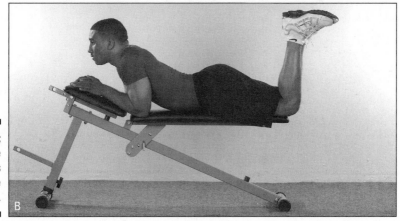

Figure 10-7:
Contract the
hamstrings
during the
up position.

Chapter 11

Buns Voyage!

• •

• •

*Y*our buns carry a lot of weight, and I'm not talking about the extra pounds you may have accumulated on your rear end over the years. Rather, your butt muscles are actually important, in a cheeky sort of way. Squeezing your bun cheeks is instrumental in lifting the rest of your body off the couch, chair, or the bleachers at a baseball game. You basically depend on your rear to get into gear. In addition, strengthening your tush now can help you avoid hip and lower-back injuries, thus keeping you mobile long into your later years.

Both men and women strive for sculpted, strong, and firm buns. However, your genetics and motivation determine your success in reaching your firming goals. (See Chapter 2 for how your body type affects realistic buns goals. You can also find several tips to get and stay motivated.) Plus, check out exercises in this chapter for buns that are strong, shapely, and firm.

Getting to Know Your Buns

Here is how your buns break down:

> ✔ When I was in college studying the names of muscles and what they did, the butt muscle always caused a few giggles. It is called the *gluteus maximus,* and I mean *maximus.* The name is perfect since it's such a large lower body muscle that stretches across your entire butt. It's the

gluteus maximus that helps you to straighten your legs to lift off a chair or get out of bed. When gym rats are referring to your butt cheek muscles, they often just call them the *glutes* (Figure 11-1 displays the gluteus maximus).

✔ Just opposite the gluteus maximus is a group of muscles called the **hip flexors.** The hip flexors are used when you kick your leg up high, use the stairs, or any time you raise your legs upward.

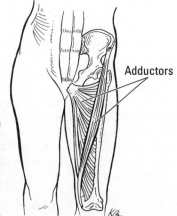

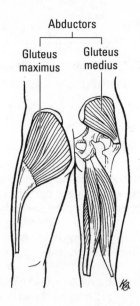

Abductors

Gluteus maximus

Gluteus medius

Adductors

Figure 11-1:
The gluteus maximus defines your butt.

Buns Exercise Techniques

Men and women constantly ask me for my secrets to a tight tush. Knowing the following basic techniques can help you get the fastest results:

✔ **Warm-up and stretch:** Do an aerobic warm-up before beginning your butt exercises. Include stretching after your exercise session (see Chapter 4 for some great lower body stretches).

✔ **Avoid holding your breath:** Exhale during exertion or when the move is most difficult.

✔ **Use the Quarter Butt Squeeze move:** While doing every butt exercise in this chapter, use what I've coined the Quarter Butt Squeeze move. Simply contract (squeeze) your butt muscles as if you were holding a quarter between your cheeks. This makes your butt exercises more effective. Try doing this squeeze throughout the day. The muscle contraction gives your butt cheeks a workout even when you are sitting. Now that makes sense.

✔ **Press your weight into your heels:** When doing butt exercises, press your weight purposely into the heels of your feet rather than into the balls of your toes. If your weight is pressed into the balls of your feet, the movement concentrates more on the quadriceps rather than the butt.

✔ **Keep your knees and toes lined up:** During butt exercises, do not let your knees extend over your toes. This can cause injury to the joint.

Reflection on hip flexion

Throughout this book, I stress the importance of balancing your body through your workout. For example, if you strengthen your chest, don't forget to work your back. If you strengthen your quads, remember to work the hamstrings, inner and outer thighs, and so on. One would think that because the hip flexors are located opposite your buns in front of your hips that you would need to work them, too. They actually are already pretty strong. In fact, working them till they are tighter than other muscles could throw your body off kilter and cause back pain. Does this mean you should forget about hip flexion? I think not!

The secret to creating that beautiful equilibrium we strive for between our buns and hips is to include plenty of hip flexion stretching in your program. This can provide a good foundation for long-term stability and flexibility in your lower body. Stretching your hip flexors may not make jaws drop when you make your entrance at a party, but it will help you look smooth as you gyrate on the dance floor and mingle cheerfully through the crowd with less or no lower back pain. (See Chapter 4 for some basic lower body stretches.) If you have extremely tight hip flexors and are looking for more stretching moves, pick up a copy of *Yoga For Dummies* or *Pilates For Dummies* (Wiley Publishing). Both are filled with great stretching moves, including hip flexion.

Kick Butt!

This exercise works to strengthen and shape the butt muscles. It also firms the backs of your thighs.

If you have back trouble, you may choose to avoid this move. (See Chapter 1 where I address medical health and safety issues.)

Getting set

Lie on the floor on your stomach. Place your head comfortably on top of your folded arms. Contract your abdominals and stretch your legs out behind you (see Figure 11-2A). Don't arch your back, it puts pressure on the spine.

The exercise

Lift your legs with flexed feet slightly off the floor. Click your heels together rapidly for ten little movements (see Figure 11-2B). Return your legs to start. This is one repetition. Do five to ten repetitions. As you progress, work up to 10 to 20 repetitions.

Do not try to lift your legs up high. This exercise is made effective by the contraction of your butt muscles to lift and squeeze your heels together, and *not* by the height of your legs.

Other options

Make it easier: Reduce the repetitions. If you cannot complete one repetition, there are plenty of other effective butt moves in this chapter that you can do instead.

Make is harder: Hold the last contraction of a repetition for a moment before returning to start.

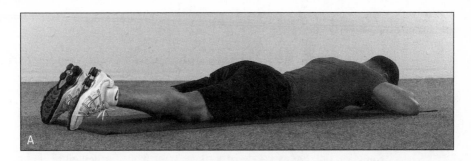

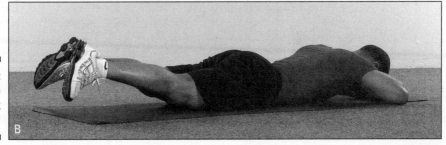

Figure 11-2:
This move
can Kick
Butt!

Floor Butt Lift

This effective exercise works to strengthen and tone the butt muscles as well as the hamstrings.

Getting set

Kneel on one leg as you gently place your front body weight on your forearms for support. Bring the opposite leg with bent knee under your chest (see Figure 11-3A). Holding the abs in tight gives you more control for the entire move.

The exercise

Fully extend your working leg from under your chest straight out behind you and slightly up (see Figure 11-3B). Slowly return to start. Do five to ten repetitions on each side. As you progress, work up to 10 to 20 repetitions on each side.

Do not arch your back or try to lift your leg up high, because that can put stress on your spine. The movement should come from contracting your butt cheeks to extend your leg.

Exhale when you extend your leg to the back. Inhale as you return it to your chest.

Other options

Hold the contraction: During the last part of the leg movement, hold the contraction for an entire two seconds to intensify the exercise.

Add ankle weights: Up the challenge of the move with ankle weights.

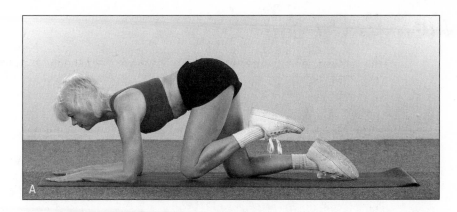

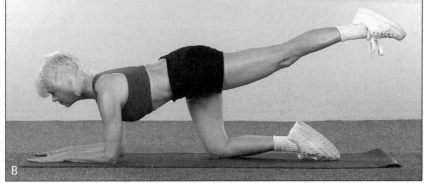

Figure 11-3:
Squeeze
your butt
cheeks
during this
move.

Bottoms Up Butt Lift

This classic exercise targets the tush. It's a move I've used many times when traveling. It can be done easily within the space constraints of a hotel room. (See Chapter 20 for more ways to fit fitness in when traveling.)

Getting set

Lie on your back with knees bent up toward the ceiling and feet flat on the floor shoulder-width apart. Rest your arms along the side of your body with palms facing down (see Figure 11-4A).

Do not arch your back. Keep your spine in neutral alignment, which means each vertebrae is elongated to lengthen your body. (See Chapter 1 for posture tips.) Hold your abs in tight throughout the move.

The exercise

Slowly contract (squeeze) your butt cheeks to lift your hips off the floor as far as is comfortable (see Figure 11-4B). Return to start. Do five to ten repetitions. As you progress, work up to 10 to 20 repetitions. Keep your neck and shoulders relaxed so as not to injure the joint.

Exhale as you lift your buttocks up. Inhale as you return to start.

Other options

Emphasize one side: For a change of pace, try swinging your weight over to one cheek during the lifting part of the exercise. Return to start and then swing your weight over to the opposite side.

Hold the contraction: Hold the contraction in the up position for a count of four. This makes the exercise more challenging.

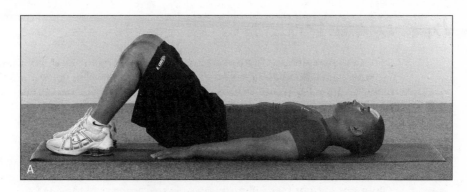

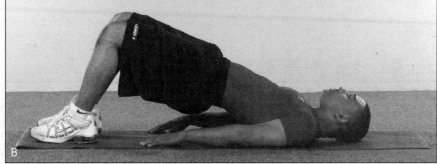

Figure 11-4:
The
Bottoms Up
Lift needs
no
equipment.

Bun Blast Off

The Bun Blast Off is a big timesaver. This one exercise works your buns, quads, hams, and inner and outer thighs, as well as your calves.

Getting set

Stand with your feet hip-width apart and knees slightly bent. Place your hands on your hips. Your toes should be pointed out slightly to the side. Hold your abs in tight (see Figure 11-5A).

Keep your upper body straight. Do not lean too far forward from the waist.

The exercise

Squat down until your thighs are parallel to the floor. Jump straight up and land on your flat feet slightly wider apart than they were at the start. Continue to squat down again until your thighs are parallel to the floor (see Figure 11-5B). Jump back to the start position. Do five to ten repetitions. As you progress, work up to 10 to 20 repetitions. Beginners should keep their hands on their hips throughout the entire exercise. Advanced exercisers can use their hands to jump up as if shooting a basket. However, be sure to keep the upper body straight.

Never let your knees extend beyond your toes so as not to injure the joint.

Other options

Do standard squats: If this is too difficult of a move, or if your knees are hurting, do the standard squats in this chapter (see next move).

Use handheld weights: Increase the difficulty of this exercise by holding a dumbbell in each hand. Your arms should be down at your side.

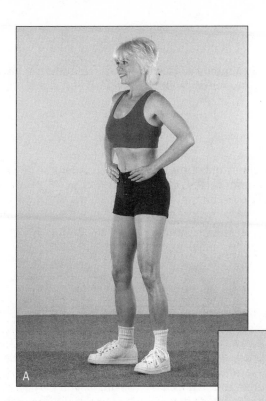

Figure 11-5:
The Bun
Blast Off is a
blast!

Squats

If you want great buns in a minimal amount of time, this move is for you. Experts rate it high. It also works the thighs.

Getting set

Stand tall with your feet hip-width apart. Your arms should be down with palms resting on top of your thighs (see Figure 11-6A).

Hold your abs in tight and butt tucked under. Elongate the spine from head to toes. (See Chapter 1 for posture tips.)

The exercise

With bent knees, slowly squat or lower your body down as you reach your arms out in front of you up to shoulder level. Stop squatting when your thighs are parallel to the floor (see Figure 11-6B). Slowly return to start. Do five to ten repetitions. As you progress, work up to 10 to 20 repetitions.

Pretend that you're sitting down in a chair. This helps you perfect the move. Remember to stop to avoid falling down! Push your weight into your heels rather than the toes. This emphasizes the butt muscles instead of the quads. Try this neat "test" — it really works! See if you can wiggle your toes in your shoes while performing your squats. If you can't, you are putting too much weight on the balls of your feet and not enough on your heels. Shift your weight accordingly.

Other options

Use a chair: If you are a beginner, place a chair behind you. Sit back into the chair briefly for support before you return to start. Be careful not to rock back and forth during this move. Doing so uses momentum rather than muscle. Momentum does nothing for the butt.

Use weights: Beef up this butt move by holding a dumbbell in each hand. Keep your arms at your side for the entire exercise.

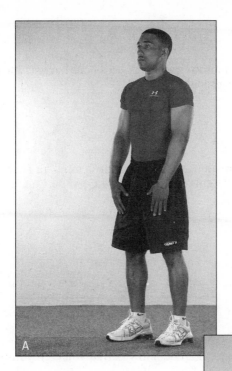

Figure 11-6:
Do squats
for hot buns
fast!

Anytime Standing Bun Burner

This exercise gets a big thumbs up from me. I do it constantly throughout the day. It lifts and tones the butt muscles.

Getting set

Whether you are cleaning, working, or playing, take a moment to stand tall and straight for this exercise. Hold your abs in tight and butt tucked under (see Figure 11-7A).

The exercise

Slowly contract and squeeze your tush to lift your leg up straight behind you (see Figure 11-7B). Slowly return to start. Do five to ten repetitions on one leg. As you progress, work up to 10 to 20 repetitions on one leg. Be sure to repeat on the opposite side.

Do not swing your leg up so high up behind you that you arch your back. This could injure the spine.

Other options

Hold the contraction: To intensify this exercise, hold the contraction for a count of four before returning to start.

Use ankle weights: Using ankle weights can give you more of a challenge.

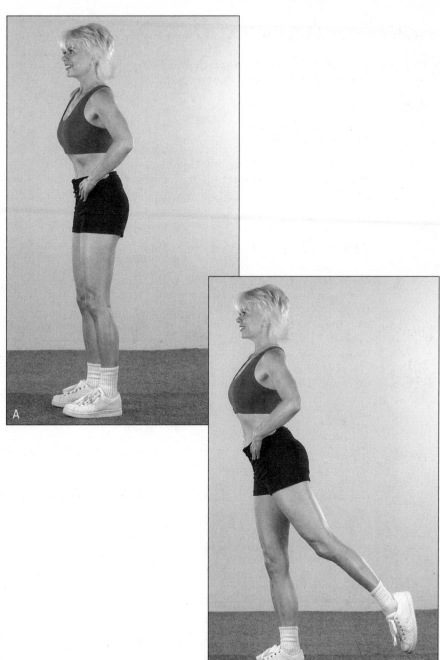

Figure 11-7:
Contract
(squeeze)
your butt
during this
move.

Chapter 12

To Calf or to Calf Not

*W*hether you are world-renowned cyclist Lance Armstrong, a member of the Riverdance cast, or simply need to tiptoe past a sleeping baby, your calf muscles play a key role in your life. And each of us can improve the strength in our calves. To achieve your personal best calf shape and strength, check out the exercises in this chapter . . . until the calves come home.

Getting to Know Your Calves

You can gain an appreciation for the strength and purpose of your calves just by checking them out in Figure 12-1. Coupled with your shin muscle, your calves are made up of the following three major lower leg muscles:

✔ **Gazing at the gastrocnemius:** The largest calf muscle in the back of your leg is called the *gastrocnemius,* which looks like a salmon fillet. However, there is nothing fishy about this powerful muscle. It helps you stand on your toes more times than you realize throughout the day. Many clients have thanked me profusely for incorporating it into their programs. One is a professional basketball player who swears that these exercises help him push off the balls of his feet for a higher and more forceful jump shot. Some of my female clients are delighted that they can now wear high heels to a special event and show off their strong and shapely gastrocnemius.

✔ **Saluting the soleus:** The second muscle of the calf is called the *soleus*. It lies underneath the gastrocnemius. The soleus works along with the gastrocnemius to lift your heels from a seated position when you press your toes into the floor.

✔ **Tracking the tibialis anterior:** The front of your lower leg is covered with a shin muscle called the *tibialis anterior.* The tibialis anterior works any time you flex your foot to press your heels into the floor.

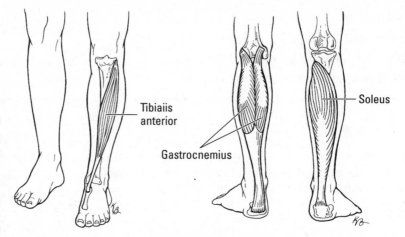

Tibiaiis anterior

Gastrocnemius

Soleus

Figure 12-1:
Check out how your calf muscles relate to each other.

Calf Exercise Techniques

Speed up the results of your calf routine with these terrific tips:

✔ **Warm-up and stretch:** Always begin your calf workout with an aerobic warm-up. It's important to stretch after a calf session. (See Chapter 4 for aerobic warm-up and specific calf-stretching moves.)

✔ **Breathe properly:** Exhale during the point of exertion when doing a calf exercise. This point occurs during the most challenging part of the movement.

✔ **Work the entire lower body:** Strong and defined calves are goals worth striving for. You can escalate the process by recognizing that they work in conjunction with the rest of your lower body. Including moves for the thighs, quads, hams, and buns creates a better equilibrium than just working the calves would, helps the calves function more efficiently, and prevents injury. (See Chapters 9, 10, and 11 for other lower body moves. For a complete custom-made leg workout, see Chapters 17 and 18.)

✔ **Avoid bouncing your calves:** It is best to do calf exercises slowly. Bouncing up and down can create painful tightness in the calf muscles.

✔ **Adjust your toe angle:** When doing a calf exercise adjust your toe angle to a point where it's comfortable. Avoid stretching the toes so far inward or outward that you place stress on the knee or ankles, causing injury.

Shying away from shin splints

Shin splints refers to a condition when the shin muscle at the front of your lower leg slightly separates away from the bone. OUCH! It can be *very* painful. The cause is usually a result of trying to do too many exercises too soon or performing a new fitness activity with too much zeal.

If you develop shin splints, try to stop the exercise temporarily for a few days. Using ice on the injury is also a good way to treat acute phases of shin splints. When the pain no longer persists, take your time getting back into the swing of things.

You can prevent shin splints by creating a workout that balances the shin and calf muscles (try the standing calf exercise in this chapter to gain lower leg harmony), changing workout shoes often to keep the shins protected with cushioning, and by avoiding running on hard surfaces such as hard concrete. If shin splints persist, talk to your doctor about possibly getting a pair of shoe inserts called orthotics.

Seated Calf Strengthener

This move works the calves to improve their shape and strength, and you'll notice an improvement in tons of everyday activities: You'll walk faster, climb steps easier, and be able to sprint to catch a phone or falling vase. All you'll need is a tubular resistance band with handles. Several manufacturers make them, such as Spri. (See Chapter 3 for more on equipment.)

Getting set

Sit on the floor and hold one handle of the tubular band in each hand. With legs outstretched in front of you, place the center of the tubing around the ball of your left, flexed foot. Bend your right knee and leg so that your right foot is flat on the floor for support. Hold your arms next to your sides. Bend the elbows and keep them next to your waist (see Figure 12-2A).

It's important to sit up tall for this exercise. Do not arch your back. Opt to elongate the spine from the tip of your head to your lower back. (See Chapter 1 for proper posture pointers.)

The exercise

Contract (squeeze) your left calf muscle as you point your left toes forward. Use your arms to tug the tubing back enough to create resistance (see Figure 12-2B). Hold for a moment and slowly return to start. Do five to ten repetitions. As you progress, work up to 10 to 20 repetitions. Repeat on the other leg.

Do not lock the knee of the working leg. Keep it slightly bent to avoid joint injury.

Other options

Increase the resistance: Tightening the grip around the handles to shorten the length of the band increases the resistance, making it a more difficult move.

Hold the contraction: Hold the contraction of the working leg for a slow count of four before returning to start. This makes the move more effective.

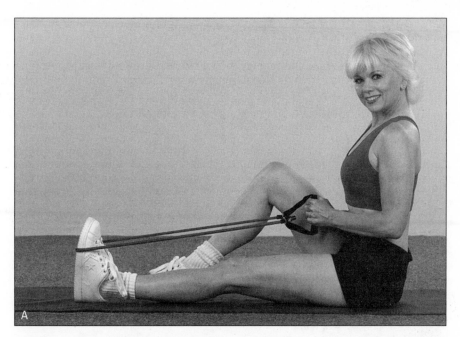

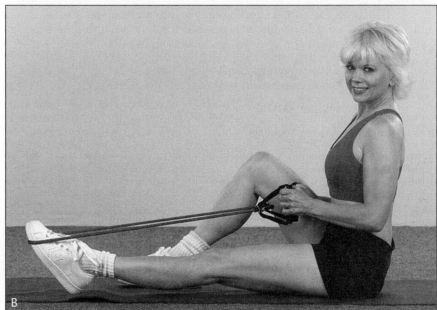

Figure 12-2:
Strengthen
calves with
this tubular
move.

Seated Calf Lift

Strengthen and tone your calves from this seated position. You need a workout bench or chair, a barbell, and a step bench. If you don't have a step bench, a raised platform or a couple of phone books will do just fine. (See Chapter 3 for more fitness equipment info.)

Getting set

Sit at the end of a workout bench. Rest your feet on top of a raised platform. Hold a barbell on top of your knees for support. Press your heels as low down as they can go (see Figure 12-3A).

Hold your head up high. Sit tall and straight, but without arching your back. Keep your abdominals tight (Chapter 1 has more information on posture).

The exercise

Lift your heels back up so that your weight is up on the balls of your feet. Hold for a moment (see Figure 12-3B). Return to start. Do five to ten repetitions. As you progress, work up to 10 to 20 repetitions.

Exhale when you lift your heels up. Inhale as you return to start.

Other options

Do it anywhere: Incorporate this move into your everyday life. Sometimes in my office, I grab something like a UPS package to rest my feet on. While talking on the phone, I define my calves. You can use no weight, which is easier, or rest several books on your lap to increase the resistance. Some parents I know work the calves while holding children.

Increase the resistance: Use more weight to make this exercise more difficult.

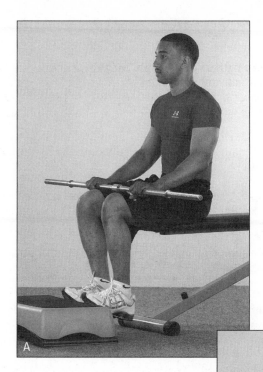

Figure 12-3:
Hold the calf
contraction
while on the
balls of your
feet.

Standing Calf

Improve the tone and strength of your calves with this move.

Getting set

Stand tall with your feet planted on the floor. Hold onto the back of a chair for support (see Figure 12-4A).

Imagine a string holding you up from your head to your feet. Keep the spine straight, abs in tight, and butt tucked under. (Check out Chapter 1 for helpful posture information.)

The exercise

Slowly lift your heels off the floor so that your weight is on the balls of your feet. Maintain proper posture. Hold for a moment (see Figure 12-4B). Return to start. Do 5 to 10 repetitions, progressing up to 10 to 20 repetitions.

Other options

Use a raised platform: To increase the difficulty, perform this move on a raised platform or a raised step. At the start, your heels should be extended as low to the floor as is possible.

Wear ankle weights: For more of a challenge, wear ankle weights to increase the resistance.

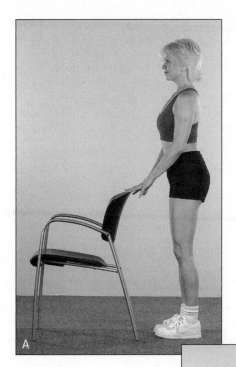

Figure 12-4:
Build
muscle with
the
Standing
Calf.

Standing Calf with Barbell

This exercise builds and strengthens the calves. It requires a considerable amount of balance, which you can achieve by having a strong core. (The exercises in Chapters 13 through 16 can aid in reaching that goal.) You need a barbell and a step bench. If you don't have a step bench, any raised platform or low step is fine. (See Chapter 3 for an explanation of this equipment.)

Getting set

Place a barbell on your shoulder. Stand tall on a raised platform or a low step. Press your heels as low as you can toward the floor (see Figure 12-5A).

Do not lock your knees. Keep them slightly bent to prevent joint injury.

Stand erect throughout the entire movement. (See Chapter 1 for good posture pointers.)

The exercise

Slowly lift your heels up till your weight is on the balls of your feet, as high as is possible without losing balance (see Figure 12-5B). Hold for a moment. Return to start. Do five to ten repetitions. As you progress, work up to 10 to 20 repetitions.

Other options

Don't use weight: Simplify this exercise by negating the resistance. It's safer to complete the move with proper technique than to wobble with too much weight.

Increase the resistance: For more of a challenge, add more weight. Remember not to arch your back or lean forward to compensate for the added resistance.

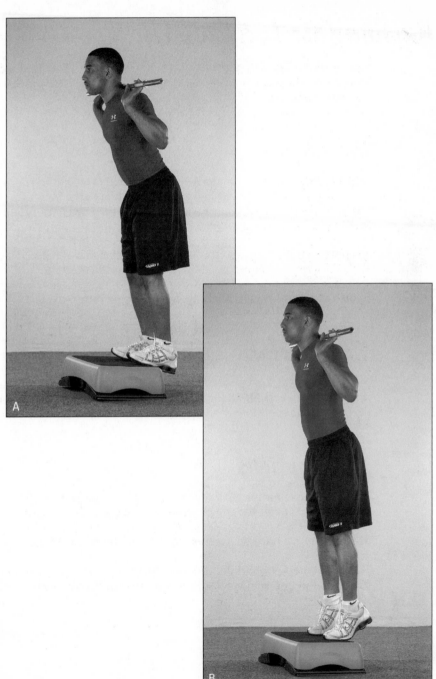

Figure 12-5:
Stand up for
your calves.

Raising One Leg Calf Lift

The One Leg Calf Lift sculpts and strengthens the calf. You need a chair for support, a raised platform or low step, and a dumbbell. (Chapter 3 discusses exercise equipment.)

Getting set

Stand on your right leg on a raised platform with a weight in your right hand down at your side. Your left hand should hold on to the back of a chair for support. Bend your left knee to lift the left leg up. Lower your right heel as low as you can to the floor (see Figure 12-6A).

Keep your spine elongated throughout the move, abs in tight, and butt tucked under. (For more on posture, check out Chapter 1.)

Exhale as you raise your heels up. Inhale as you return to start.

The exercise

Slowly lift the heel of your right working leg till your weight is on the ball of your foot. Pause and hold for a moment (see Figure 12-6B). Return to start. Do five to ten repetitions. As you progress, work up to 10 to 20 repetitions.

Other options

Make the move easier: Simplify this exercise by not using weight. You can always add on more resistance when you get stronger.

Make the move harder: Add resistance to increase the difficulty of the move.

Hold the contraction: Hold the calf contraction in the up position for a count of four before returning to start to increase the effectiveness of the move.

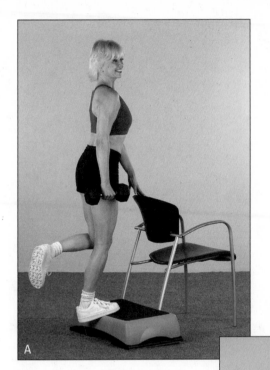

Figure 12-6:
Stand tall
during this
exercise.

Part IV
Core: Abs and Lower Back

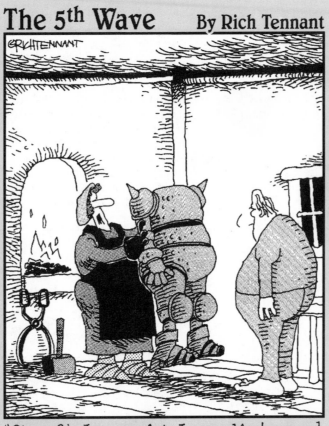

The 5th Wave   By Rich Tennant

"Okay, Sir Loungealot, I was able to pound out another inch in the waist, but you're gonna have to start taking care of yourself or buy a new suit of armor."

In this part . . .

If you covet fabulous abs and a trim waistline, then this part is for you. You can discover lots of no-nonsense exercise to shape up your entire midsection. With these moves, you can define every segment of your abdominal muscles, including obliques, lower abs, and upper abs. There's also a whole chapter chock-full of lower-back exercises to stabilize your core area and enhance the results of your abs work. In a crunch? This part is for you!

Chapter 13

Peak Obliques

. . . .

In This Chapter

▶ Discovering how the oblique muscles work

▶ Improving your oblique workout technique

▶ Getting into oblique exercises

. . . .

*Y*our *oblique* muscles — your side abdominals — are responsible for a number of activities. When you bend from the side or twist to reach something behind you, the oblique muscles are contracting. Strong obliques add support to the lower back, warding off back pain and posture problems and ultimately promoting increased stability. Plus, your improved posture, made possible through strong obliques, gives your figure a slimming effect. So to improve your posture and tone those obliques, check out the great moves in this chapter.

Getting to Know Your Obliques

Your abdominals consist of four muscles. Most people are used to hearing them simply called *abs*. The abs include the *Rectus abdominis,* the *Transversus abdominis,* and a pair of muscles called the *obliques* (see Figure 13-1). This chapter concentrates on the obliques. (Refer to Chapters 14 and 15 for more on the other abdominal muscle groups.)

The oblique muscles actually include the following pair of muscles on each of your sides:

  ✔ The *external obliques* form the top muscle.

  ✔ The *internal obliques* lie underneath the external obliques.

Together, they cross diagonally near the side of your midsection, from the bottom of your rib cage to your pubic area (see Figure 13-1). The obliques are responsible for side bending and waist twisting moves.

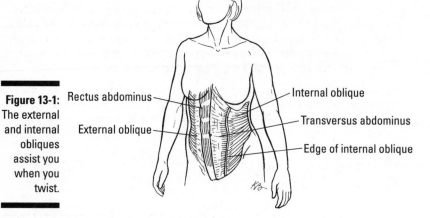

Figure 13-1: Rectus abdominus — Internal oblique
The external
and internal — External oblique — Transversus abdominus
obliques — Edge of internal oblique
assist you
when you
twist.

Oblique Exercise Techniques

Because doing oblique exercises properly can speed up your results, whereas doing them improperly can turn working out your waist into a waste of time, follow these tips:

- ✔ **Warm-up and stretch:** Including an aerobic warm-up as well as stretching after your workout are essential for success. (See Chapter 4.)

- ✔ **Breathe properly:** Exhale during the exertion part of an exercise. Usually, that's the most difficult part of a move. Don't worry about any confusing mumbo jumbo. For all of the exercises in this chapter, simply blow the air out when you lift your upper torso up off the floor.

- ✔ **Use quality versus quantity:** Somewhere along the way, fitness enthusiasts began to replace the quality of an oblique move with quantity. Somehow it became important to do hundreds of oblique repetitions with no attention given to proper form. This is erroneous. It is far better to do 8 to 20 repetitions with the correct form that I describe than to do numerous but sloppy moves.

- ✔ **Lift from your obliques:** When doing these side oblique exercises, don't lift from your neck. Doing so could cause injury and does absolutely nothing for your waistline. The lift comes from your obliques.

- ✔ **Keep your chin up:** Keep your chin slightly up throughout oblique exercises to avoid neck injury. Imagine holding an orange under your chin during the moves to ensure proper form.

✔ **Avoid thinking you can just zap them:** As you embark on your awesome obliques journey, keep in mind that you cannot spot reduce. Shrinking your waist size is an attainable goal *if*, in addition to doing the exercises in this chapter, you maintain a healthy diet and include a cardiovascular activity in your routine. (Review Chapter 2 where I address how you can replace fat from your waistline with firm oblique muscles.)

✔ **Maintain a neutral spine:** In past years, fitness experts harped at clients to push their backs into the floor during oblique moves. This was good advice in that it is harmful to arch the back during abdominal exercises. However, it does not allow for the natural curve of the spine. The best current advice is not to arch *or* flatten the back. It is safest to keep a small distance of about an inch and a half between your back and the floor, which varies slightly depending on what's comfortable for you.

Trashing a waist-ful move

Working out the obliques is sure to tone your waist quickly. However, there is a popular exercise that I wish would disappear because it is of no benefit. Many people do side bends with a weight in each hand. They swing side to side in an effort to slim the sides. This bending move is useless and in fact could build a *wider* waist. Throw it out! Opt for the peak oblique moves in this chapter. Custom-make an individualized program that works your obliques and other core muscles from the ready-to-go fitness menus in Chapters 17 and 18.

Oblique Crunch

This Oblique Crunch concentrates on both the external and internal obliques.

Getting set

Lie on your back with your hands behind your head so that your fingers rest behind your ears. Open your elbows up and out to the side. Keep your shoulder blades on the floor. Lift your knees up and together as you bring them to one side. Keep them stacked on top of each other (see Figure 13-2A).

The exercise

Using slow and controlled movements, raise your upper torso directly off the floor. Contract or crunch your rib cage in the direction of your pelvis (see Figure 13-2B). Slowly return to start. Do five to ten repetitions on each side. As you progress, work up to 10 to 20 repetitions on each side.

Be sure to keep your chin up as if you are holding an orange. This will help to prevent neck injury.

Exhale as you lift your upper torso toward your pelvis. Inhale on the return to start.

Other options

Cross your arms: If the Oblique Crunch is too difficult, you can do the same move with your arms crossed over your chest. Be extra careful to keep your chin up to avoid neck injury.

Use a stability ball: To take the Oblique Crunch to an advanced level, try using a stability ball. (See Chapter 3 for more information on equipment.) The move is slightly different, but it works the same muscles. Place the ball on the floor near a wall. Lie sideways on the ball with your hands behind your head. Push the bottoms of your feet into the wall to help you stabilize yourself. It may take practice to achieve balance. Lift your upper torso as you crunch to the side toward your hip. Return to start. This is a challenging move so only do it if you can maintain proper form throughout.

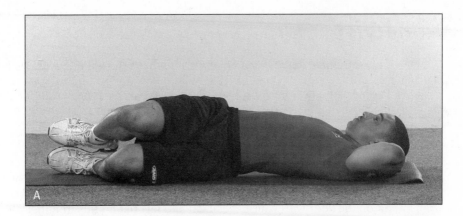

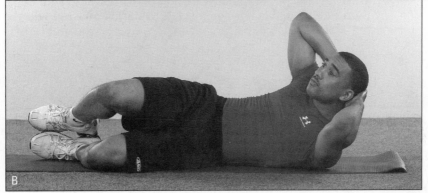

Figure 13-2:
Slow, controlled movements enhance the Oblique Crunch.

Side Twist

This rotational move tones up and strengthens the oblique muscles.

People with lower back problems should avoid this type of rotational movement. The Lift and Cross exercise in this chapter may be a better choice for you.

Getting set

Sit on the floor with your knees bent and feet flat on the ground. Hold your arms out directly in front of you over your knees. Lean your upper back backward enough so that it is comfortable to start at a 45- to 60-degree angle to the floor (see Figure 13-3A).

The exercise

Not reaching up higher than 45 to 60 degrees from the floor, rotate and stretch to one side (see Figure 13-3B). Without stopping, rotate to the other side. Keep alternating until you complete five to ten repetitions on each side. As you progress, work up to 10 to 20 repetitions on each side.

Do not arch your back. It helps to hold your head up high and chin raised. The rotation should be smooth and controlled — no jerky movements.

Exhale as you shift to each side. Inhale on the return toward the center.

Other options

Secure your feet: Placing your feet under an object such as a bed or sofa makes the movement simpler. Ask a friend to hold your feet down.

Place your hands behind your head: For more of a challenge, place your hands behind your head, and, as you make the rotation move, lead with your shoulder rather than with your elbow. Keep the elbows open and out to the side for the entire exercise.

Use a stability ball: Using a stability ball turns the Side Twist into an advanced exercise. (See Chapter 3 for more on equipment.) Maintain balance on the ball as you complete the Side Twist move. In addition to the obliques, other core muscles spring into action.

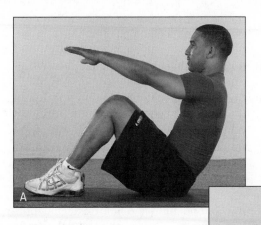

Figure 13-3:
Rotation
strengthens
the
obliques.

Elbow to Knee

This exercise emphasizes the external obliques.

Getting set

Lie on your back on the floor with your feet flat on the ground and your hands behind your head. Your fingers should be gently resting behind your ears, and your elbows should be opened and out to the side (see Figure 13-4A).

Keep your spine in an elongated position and neutral alignment throughout the entire exercise — do not arch your back or keep it flat. (Review Chapter 1 for more on proper posture.) Keep your neck straight and chin raised up.

The exercise

At the same time that you raise your right leg up and kick it out straight in front of you, lift your right shoulder, and then bring your right elbow toward your left raised knee. Keep your left upper arm lightly pressed into the floor for support. You should feel the contraction or squeeze on the upper right side of your abs or external obliques (see Figure 13-4B). Hold for a count of four and return to start. Repeat on other side. Do 5 to 10 repetitions alternating on each side, working up to 10 to 20 repetitions alternating on each side.

You have probably seen fitness enthusiasts at the gym swinging elbows back and forth faster than a propeller. Sorry to say — they may be working hard, but they are hardly working. You can avoid this dilemma by not pulling your neck with your hands. To effectively complete this exercise, the lift should come from raising your shoulder through the contraction of your obliques. The elbow merely assists in this action.

Exhale as you lift up to contract your obliques. Inhale as you return to start.

Other options

Cross your chest: To simplify this exercise, keep your arms crossed over your chest throughout the move. Keep your head and chin raised up.

Hold a weight: To increase the difficulty, hold a weight in your hands over your chest throughout the move. Be sure that you maintain the correct form that I describe in the exercise. (Refer to Chapter 3 where I explain how to increase weight safely.)

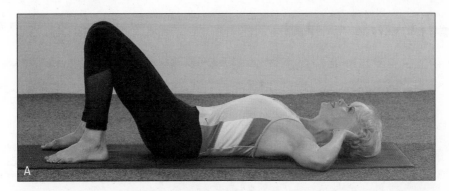

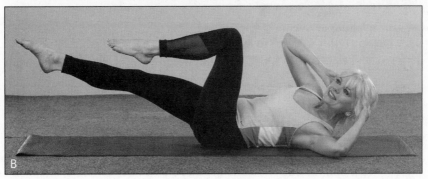

Figure 13-4:
This move
strengthens
the
obliques,
especially
the external
ones.

Lift and Cross

This rotation exercise gives your obliques a superb workout.

Getting set

Lie on the floor on your back so that your knees are bent and your feet are flat on the floor. Your hands should be behind your head so that your fingers rest on the backs of your ears. Keep your elbows open and outward (see Figure 13-5A).

Neither arch your back nor keep it flat. You should maintain an elongated spine throughout the exercise. Keep the chin up and your neck lengthened and straight. (See Chapter 1 for good posture information.)

The exercise

Slowly lift your left shoulder up toward your right knee. Do not lift your knee up for this variation of the exercise (see Figure 13-5B). Contract your abdominals and then slowly return to start. Do five to ten repetitions on each side. As you progress, do 10 to 20 repetitions on each side.

You may want to bend your elbow as you cross to the opposite side, but don't. Keep your elbows open and use the obliques to lift the shoulder.

Exhale as you lift your upper torso up and inhale as you return to start.

Other options

Lift your legs: To make this exercise easier, lift your legs up so that they rest at a 90-degree angle on a sofa or stool. Complete the move as described.

Lift your knee: To add a bit of a challenge, simultaneously lift your opposite knee toward your shoulder.

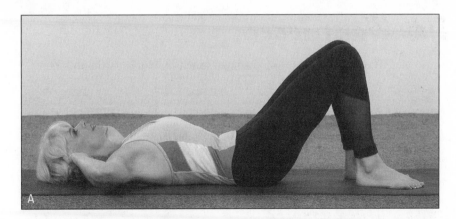

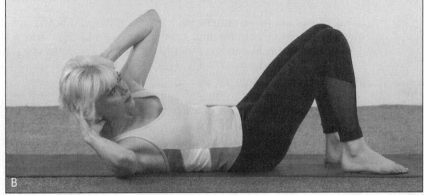

Figure 13-5:
Lift and
Cross to
peak
obliques.

Side Waist Toner

This move helps to tone up the waist by working the obliques.

Getting set

Lie on your back with your knees bent and feet flat on the floor. Rest your arms along the sides of your body (see Figure 13-6A).

The exercise

Slowly raise your torso and lift your left shoulder and both arms up and toward the outside of your right knee (see Figure 13-6B). Make a tiny pulsating contraction for five to ten repetitions. Slowly return to start. Repeat on the other side. Do two sets. As you progress, work up to two sets of 10 to 20 repetitions on each side.

Exhale as you lift your torso up. Continue to breathe throughout the pulsating action. Inhale as you return to start.

Other options

Lift your feet: Elevating your feet on a sofa or chair so that your legs form a 90-degree angle is easier than the original move.

Extend your legs up: Raising and extending your legs up straight toward the ceiling creates an advanced version of the exercise. Do not bend your neck and head. Keep the chin raised up.

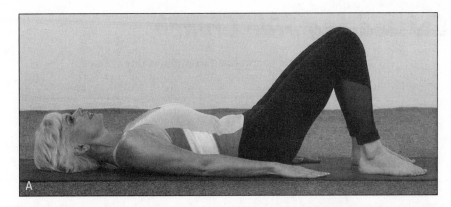

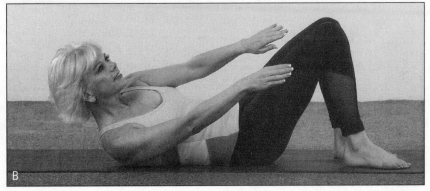

Figure 13-6:
Tone up
your waist
with this
move.

Crossed Leg Side Crunch

This exercise hones in on the oblique muscles.

Getting set

Lie on your back with your feet flat on the floor and knees bent up toward the ceiling. Cross the left leg over the right at your left calf. Your hands should be behind your head so that your fingers rest behind your ears. Keep your elbows open and out to the side (see Figure 13-7A).

The exercise

Keep your left elbow positioned on the floor for stability as you raise your right shoulder toward your left knee. Pause for a moment (see Figure 13-7B). Slowly return to start.

Repeat the move for two sets of five to ten repetitions. Be sure to do the opposite side. As you progress, work up to 2 sets of 10 to 20 repetitions on each side.

Do no arch your back. Use your obliques to crunch your upper torso forward and not your elbow.

Exhale as you lift your torso up. Inhale as you return to start.

Other options

Easier: Simplify by crossing the ankle of your leg at the opposite knee.

Harder: Make the move more advanced by crossing the knee of one leg over the opposite knee. Be sure to lift from the shoulder and obliques rather than with your elbow.

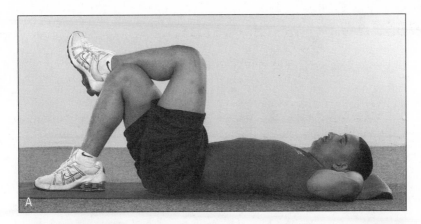

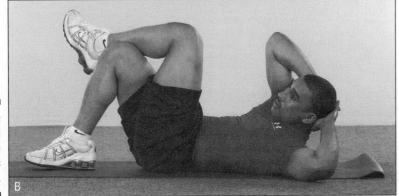

Figure 13-7:
The Crossed
Leg Side
Crunch gets
results.

Chapter 14

Bustin' that Beer Belly: Lower Abs

....

....

Both men and women struggle continuously, for obvious aesthetic reasons, to lose their flab, accusingly called a gut or beer belly. Aside from aesthetic reasons, strengthening your lower abs makes activities, such as raking leaves, picking up heavy objects, or even standing in long shopping lines, easier. By strengthening your lower abs, you can also avoid posture and back problems and you ultimately benefit from improved stability and a stronger core (your abs and lower back).

Doing lower abs movements is not enough to lose your pouch. You still must lose the excess fat in order to show off your toned muscles, which means coupling these exercises with a healthy diet and aerobic activities. (See Chapter 19 and 20 respectively.)

Getting to Know Your Lower Abs Muscles

The abdominals actually consist of four muscles: the *rectus abdominis,* the *transversus abdominis,* and the *external* and *internal obliques.* This chapter focuses on the lower muscle fibers of the rectus abdominis. Check out the following descriptions of the rectus abdominis as well as the transversus abdominis:

> ✔ **Remembering the rectus abdominis:** The *rectus abdominis* is the abdominal muscle that gets most of the attention — the famous "washboard." Although you may think it's two muscles because of the separate upper and lower abs action, it's actually one long, wide, flat muscle

that covers a large part of your middle torso from the lower chest to the pubic bone. The rectus abdominis helps you pull your rib cage toward your hips (upper abs) or your hips toward your rib cage (lower abs). (See Figure 14-1.)

✔ **Talking about the transversus abdominis:** The *transversus abdominis* lies underneath your rectus abdominis and runs horizontally across your mid-section (see Figure 14-1). It contributes to posture, balance, and stability, and you use it when you hiccup, cough, or sneeze. I love this muscle because it makes me laugh — literally. Whenever you laugh so hard that your abs hurt, that is your transversus abdominis working.

Figure 14-1:
The lower abs portion of the rectus abdominis and the transversus abdominis are highlighted.

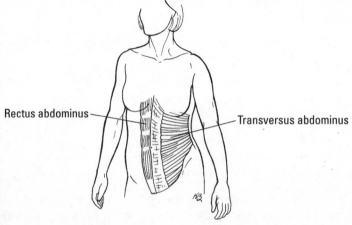

Rectus abdominus — Transversus abdominus

Lower Abs Exercise Techniques

You can bust that beer belly in a minimum amount of time if you eat a balanced diet, do aerobic activities, and use the following good lower abs exercise techniques:

✔ **Warm-up and stretch:** Include an aerobic warm-up as well as stretching after your lower abs workout. (See Chapter 4.)

✔ **Breathe properly:** Exhale at the point of exertion or, simply put, during the most difficult part of the exercise.

✔ **Avoid momentum:** Because many lower abs exercises involve raising the lower part of your stomach, it's all too easy to use momentum to complete the movement. Swinging your lower abs or legs up and down uncontrollably works with gravity but, unfortunately, does nothing to tone that belly. Your strength should come from your core (abs and lower back), not the earth's gravitational field.

- ✔ **Tighten those abs:** Remember to contract or squeeze your lower abs to get the most out of the exercises.

- ✔ **Stop the slop:** If you find that your form starts to get sloppy — stop! It's better to do fewer repetitions with correct form than to do tons of lower abs exercises with poor technique.

- ✔ **Make a mental and physical plan:** Use the power of mind over body to capitalize on your lower abs workout. (Take a look at Chapter 2 where I explain how to create a mental and physical plan that can speed up lower abs strength results.)

- ✔ **Hold the contraction:** Holding the contraction of a lower abs move is a powerful action. It completes the lifting part of the movement and makes it more effective.

Making the most of your abs

There are a number of books and tapes on the market that promise great abs. _Ten Minute Tone-Ups For Dummies_ is, naturally, a fabulous start that can carry your waistline into a trim future. However, if you are looking for other products that will complement the present volume, try my _29-Minute Tummy Toner_ video. It includes more great abs exercises that are simple, effective, and fun to do. _The 29-Minute Tummy Toner_ is distributed by Goodtimes Home Video and available at my Web site: www.starglow.com. Of course, you still need to do an aerobic activity regularly and maintain a healthy diet if you want fabulous abs. (Chapter 20 addresses the benefits of a cardiovascular workout. In Chapter 19, I discuss making smart food choices.) For more in-depth information on how to eat right and stay healthy, pick up a copy of _Nutrition For Dummies._ It's jam-packed with tips that will help you make the most of your midsection.

Lower Abs Lift

This great move strengthens and flattens your lower stomach muscles.

Getting set

Lie on your back with your legs raised and knees bent at a 90-degree angle. You are in correct form if your knees are pointing up to the ceiling and your shins are parallel to the floor. Rest your arms down by your sides (see Figure 14-2A).

Do not arch your back. Keep it in neutral alignment, meaning your spine is elongated from top to bottom, allowing for its natural curve. Keep the chin raised as if you're holding an orange under it.

The exercise

Lift your pelvis toward your rib cage by contracting the abdominals. At the same time, raise your tailbone off the floor to move your knees in the direction of your chin. Pause as you squeeze and hold your abdominals in for a moment (see Figure 14-2B). Slowly return to start. Do five to ten repetitions. As you progress, work up to 10 to 20 repetitions.

To get the most benefit out of this Lower Abs Lift move, be sure to use your abdominal muscles to lift the pelvis rather than your butt muscles. This takes sharp mind over body concentration (see Chapter 2).

Other options

Place your feet on the ground: You can simplify the move by placing your feet flat on the ground hip-width apart with your knees pointing up toward the ceiling. Use your lower abdominals to tilt your pelvis slightly up.

Use a stability ball: For more of a challenge, try it with a stability ball (see Chapter 3 for equipment information). Lie on your back on the ball so that your hips are lower than your shoulders. Raise your arms up over your head to hold onto a weighted object such as a chair for balance. Curl your legs up toward your chest. Do not hyperextend your back.

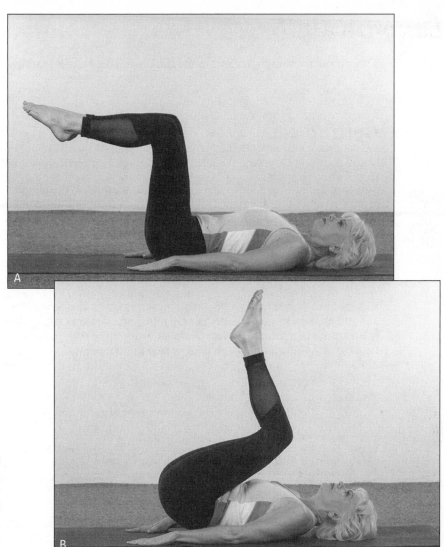

Figure 14-2:
The Lower Abs Lift targets the lower abs.

Belly Be My Best

This exercise strengthens and tones the lower abs while it stabilizes your core.

Getting set

Lie on the floor on your back with your arms outstretched to the side (see Figure 14-3A).

Do not arch your back. Keep your head against the floor. Elongate your spine from the tip of your head down to your toes.

The exercise

Slightly bend both knees as you raise both legs up to 75 degrees. Squeeze your abs and hold up to one minute. Slowly return to start. If you are starting out, do one to three repetitions. As you progress, work up to three to five repetitions (see Figure 14-3B). If time permits, feel free to do more.

Other options

Make it easier: With one knee bent, plant that foot firmly into the floor. Straighten and lift the opposite leg to a 90-degree angle with your foot flexed. Slowly lift and then lower it in one continuous motion. Repeat on the opposite leg. Do five to ten repetitions on each leg. As you progress, work up to 10 to 20 repetitions on each leg.

Make it harder: Rather than bending your knees slightly, keep the knees straight but not locked. Remember to hold the abdominals in tight.

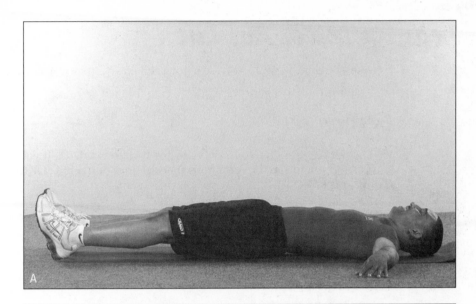

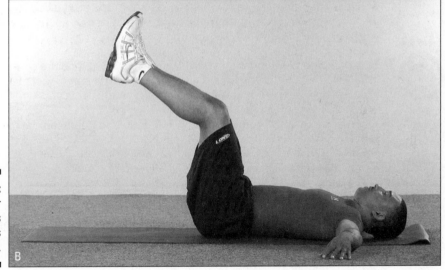

Figure 14-3:
Tighten your
lower abs
with this
move.

Legs Up Lower Abs Lift

Strengthen your lower abs with this powerful lift.

Getting set

Lie on your back so that your arms are down at your sides. Lift your legs up and point them toward the ceiling so that they are perpendicular to the floor (see Figure 14-4A).

Keep your chin up as if you are holding an orange under it. Your head should be flat on the floor and neck straight.

The exercise

Squeeze your stomach as you slightly lift your hips off the floor (see Figure 14-4B). Pause and slowly return to start. Do five to ten repetitions. As you progress, work up to 10 to 20 repetitions.

Do not let momentum swing your hips up and down. Use the contractions of your lower abs to lift the hips. This is a very subtle move — sometimes less than an inch. Keep your shoulders on the ground.

Exhale when you lift your legs up, which is the most difficult part of the move.

Other options

Do Lower Abs Lift: If this exercise leaves you rocking your butt up and down rather than lifting the lower abs, your stomach is probably not strong enough. Stick with the Lower Abs Lift exercise described earlier in this chapter until your strength is increased. Be patient!

Place your hands behind your head: To make this move more challenging, do it with your hands behind your head.

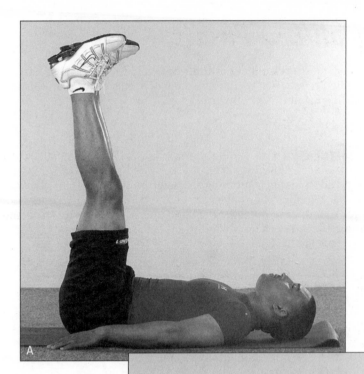

Figure 14-4:
Avoid
rocking
when
performing
the Legs Up
Lower Abs
Lift.

Tummy Pull/Leg Push

This is a great exercise that concentrates on the lower abs. At first, it may seem difficult, but after you get the hang of it, this move may become your favorite. It's fun and very effective.

Getting set

Sit on the floor so that your arms are behind you. Bend your elbows to lean slightly back so that your hands are on the floor with your fingers pointing forward. Your knees should be bent and pointing up toward the ceiling. Lift and crunch your knees up toward your chest to form the start position of this exercise (see Figure 14-5A).

The exercise

Lean slightly back again as you use your lower abs to slowly push your legs out at a 45-degree angle to the floor (see Figure 14-5B). Slowly return to the knee-to-chest start position. Do five to ten repetitions. As you progress, work up to 10 to 20 repetitions.

Don't cheat yourself by using gravity to rock back and forth. Focus on the abdominal contraction.

Breathing can be confusing with this move because the entire exercise requires exertion. Exhale when you lift or contract the lower abs, and don't hold your breath.

Other options

Do fewer repetitions: This move is challenging. If you can't do it in the correct form that I describe, don't do so many repetitions. One repetition in fine form is far better than 20 using a sloppy technique that could injure your spine.

Pause for a count: Increase the difficulty of the move by extending your legs out for a count of four before returning to start.

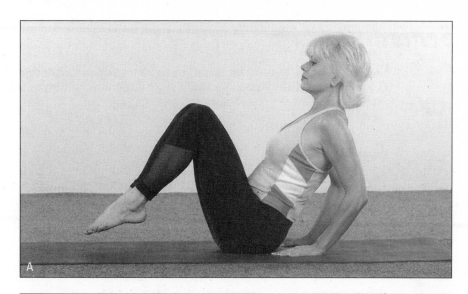

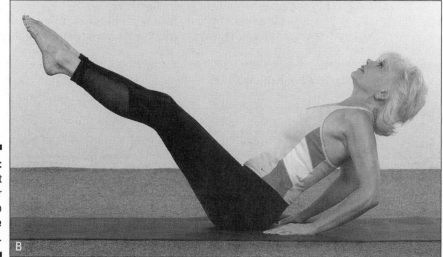

Figure 14-5:
Contract
your lower
abs to
enhance
this move.

Seated Leg Lift

I'm always on the lookout for fast-fitness moves that can be done anywhere. This efficient and very effective exercise fits the bill at no cost to you but with a big pay off — great-looking lower abs.

Getting set

This part is easy. Grab a chair from your office, dining room, living room, or anywhere. Sit tall with your feet planted on the floor. Place your hands underneath your thighs (see Figure 14-6A).

The exercise

Slowly pull your knees up toward your chest. Contract or squeeze your abdominals as you hold for a count of four (see Figure 14-6B). Slowly return to start. Do five to ten repetitions. As you progress, work up to 10 to 20 repetitions.

Check your posture during the Seated Leg Lift. Sitting does not mean that it's okay to slouch. Elongate the spine as if a puppeteer were holding you up. Do not stick your butt out or arch your back. Maintain neutral posture. (Review Chapter 1 for proper posture.)

Exhale when you lift your knees up toward your chest. Inhale when you return to start.

Other options

Seated pelvic tilt: From a seated position, use your lower abs to slightly tilt your pelvis up.

Seated tummy toner: From a seated position, hold your stomach in tight. Hold for 5 seconds and release. Remember to breathe through the contraction (squeeze).

Tummy pull/leg push: This move is an advance version of the Seated Leg Lift. Follow the description of the Tummy Pull/Leg Push that I gave earlier in this chapter, but perform the move while seated on a chair.

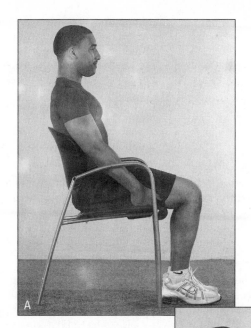

Figure 14-6:
No more
excuses!
You can
do this
lower abs
exercise
anywhere.

Bicycle

This quaint, old-fashioned exercise still does a great job of whipping your lower abs into shape.

Getting set

Lie on your back so that your head is resting on your hands with elbows bent and out to the side. Raise your upper body (head, neck, shoulders) as you pull your knees up toward your chest.

The exercise

Push your left leg out at the same time you twist your torso to bring your left elbow to the right knee (see Figure 14-7A). Return to start as you pull both knees into your chest. Without stopping, push out your right leg at the same time you twist your torso to bring your right elbow to the left knee (see Figure 14-7B). Repeat this continuous motion by alternating five times on each side. As you progress, work up to alternating ten times on each side.

Exhale when you push your legs out. Inhale when you return to the center start position.

Other options

Decrease the repetitions: Using correct form is far more important than the number of repetitions you complete. Decrease the repetitions to simplify the challenge.

Hold for a count: Increase the level of difficulty by pausing when you extend your leg out. Contract your abdominals and hold for a count of four before twisting to the other side.

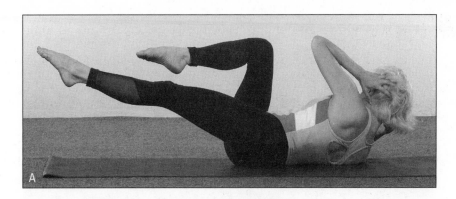

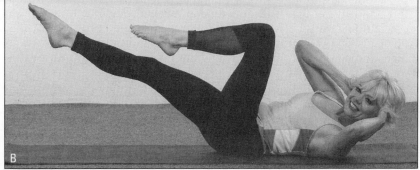

Figure 14-7:
Ride this
bicycle to
lower abs
success!

Chapter 15

Ab-Sense Makes the Waist Look Slimmer: Upper Abs

Sporting a "six-pack" — that visible washboard effect of a toned tummy — is on the wish list of many people. But strong upper abs sport health benefits also. Together with the rest of your abdominal muscles and lower back, they form what fitness experts call the *core*. The core takes the credit for supporting your lower back and stabilizing your posture for everything you do. When you walk, stand, or even sleep, the core muscles are working. Without them, your body would just collapse. Keeping them strong may even ward off back pain. To get your upper abs in good working order try out the strengthening moves in this chapter.

To what degree you can achieve those rock hard upper abs, though, depends on a number of factors, such as genetics and how willing you are to work. (To help you get and stay motivated, I provide some surefire hints in Chapter 2. I also explain how your genetic body type and muscle fiber differences can affect your results.)

Getting to Know Your Upper Abs

The abdominal muscles, more commonly called the abs, are actually made up of four muscles. Their technical names are: the *rectus abdominis, transversus abdominis,* and the *external and internal obliques* (see Figure 15-1). This chapter concentrates on the upper fibers of the rectus abdominis. (Refer to Chapters 13 and 14 for more on the other abdominal muscles.)

The rectus abdominis is actually one long, wide, flat muscle that stretches from the lower chest to the pubic bone. Many people mistakenly think of it as two muscles (upper and lower abs). Truthfully, any time you do an abdominal exercise, you work your entire rectus abdominis. However, when you lift your hips to your chest, you are concentrating on the fibers of the lower part of the rectus abdominis, and when you lift your chest toward your hips you're focusing on the fibers of the upper part of the rectus abdominis. Because the work in this chapter is primarily for the upper portion of the rectus abdominis, I will bow to convention and use the term most people call it — the *upper abs*.

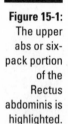
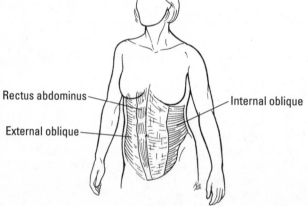

Figure 15-1:
The upper abs or six-pack portion of the Rectus abdominis is highlighted.

Rectus abdominus

Internal oblique

External oblique

Upper Abs Exercise Techniques

Speed up the results of your upper abs workout by using the following tips on proper form and technique:

- ✔ **Warm-up and stretch:** Always do an aerobic warm-up when starting your abs workout session. Include stretching after the routine. (See Chapter 4 for more on warming-up and stretching.)

- ✔ **Breathe properly:** Exhale at the most challenging part of an upper abs move (during exertion), which is when you lift your upper torso off the floor.

✔ **Don't do neck lifts:** Use your upper abs to lift your upper torso. I have seen so many people vigorously lifting their necks and heads up and down, which does nothing for the upper abs and could cause injury. Instead, keep your chin raised up as if it's holding an orange in place. Keep your head and neck steady during the whole movement.

✔ **Don't arch your back:** Keep the movement of your upper abs safe and effective with proper posture. Do not arch your back or flatten it. Keep about an inch and a half between your back and the floor. This will vary slightly depending on the natural curvature of your spine and what is comfortable for you. (See Chapter 1 for posture tips.)

✔ **Curl up:** Don't just lift your upper torso up and down during these exercises. Add an extra squeeze of the abdominal muscles, allowing you to curl up. Imagine a friend dropping a basketball on your stomach. It's that extra contraction that gets the fastest upper abs results.

Speeding up results – abs order!

The order you do your abdominal exercises in can make a difference in your results. Whether you are doing exercises for the upper abs, lower abs, or obliques, the upper abs are activated. That's why it's best to do concentrated upper abs last. If you did them first, they would get tired and not be as strong for the other abdominal exercises. Rest assured that if you mess the order up, it is not harmful. It's just not as effective. For the speediest results, follow this abs order: obliques, lower abs, upper abs. (For a choice of ready-to-go abs workout menus, check out Chapters 17 and 18, where I place the exercises in the abs order that can deliver the fastest abs results.)

Crunch

This classic move works all the abdominal muscles with a special emphasis on the upper abs.

Getting set

Lie on your back with your feet flat on the floor and knees bent pointing up toward the ceiling. Fold your arms across your chest. Hold your chin up as if you are holding an orange (see Figure 15-2A).

Do not arch your back or press it flat. Keep it in neutral alignment. (See Chapter 1 for proper posture tips.)

The exercise

Contract or squeeze your abdominal muscles to help you lift your upper torso up off the floor. When your shoulder blades are raised up, pause for a moment (see Figure 15-2B). Slowly return to start. Do five to ten repetitions. As you progress, work up to 10 to 20 repetitions.

Exhale as you lift your torso up. Inhale as you return to start.

Other options

Place your arms at your sides: Placing your arms at your sides takes the crunch to a beginner level.

Hold a weight: Holding a weight in your hand on your chest is more challenging. If you place it over your head, it is even more advanced. Make sure that you do not arch your back.

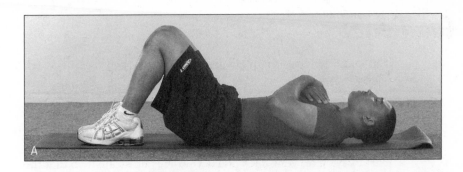

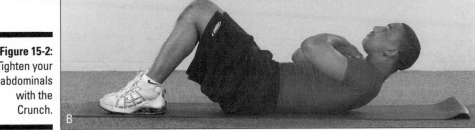

Figure 15-2:
Tighten your
abdominals
with the
Crunch.

Toe Reach

If your goal is to reach for sculpted upper abs, then the Toe Reach is definitely for you.

Getting set

Start by lying on your back. Raise your legs up straight so that they are perpendicular to the floor at a 90-degree angle. With your hands together, extend your arms up toward your feet (see Figure 15-3A).

The exercise

Contract your upper abs as you reach toward your feet. Hold the contraction for a brief moment (see Figure 15-3B). Slowly return to start. Do five to ten repetitions. As you progress, work up to 10 to 20 repetitions.

Keep the movements slow and controlled — not jerky.

Exhale as you lift up toward your toes. Inhale as you return to start.

Other options

Place your hands at your sides: Place your hands at your sides while you lift your upper torso toward your toes. This makes for an easier move. You can do this version until your upper abs become stronger.

Place your hands behind your head: This is a more advanced move. If you select this option, keep your elbows open and out to the side.

Make it an oblique move: Turn this exercise into an oblique move by reaching toward your opposite foot. Alternate sides. (For more oblique exercises, check out Chapter 13.)

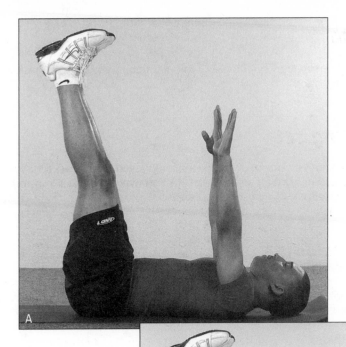

Figure 15-3:
The Toe
Reach
works the
upper abs.

Wall Reach

The Wall Reach works all the abdominal muscles with an emphasis on the upper abs.

Getting set

Start by lying on your back with your legs raised up against a wall so that they are perpendicular to the floor. Lift and extend your arms straight up toward your feet. Place your butt as close to the wall as possible (see Figure 15-4A).

The exercise

Use your upper abdominals to help you lift your upper torso toward your feet. Hold the contraction for a brief moment (see Figure 15-4B). Slowly return to start. Do five to ten repetitions. As you progress, work up to 10 to 20 repetitions.

Exhale as you lift your upper body up. Inhale as you return to start.

Avoid jerky movements. Use slow, controlled movements.

Other options

Place your hand at your sides: Place your hands at your sides while you lift your upper torso toward your toes. Doing the exercise this way makes the Wall Reach less challenging.

Keep your hands behind your head: This makes the exercise more advanced. Be sure to keep your elbows open and out to the side. Do not lace your fingers. It's best to gently rest them behind your ears.

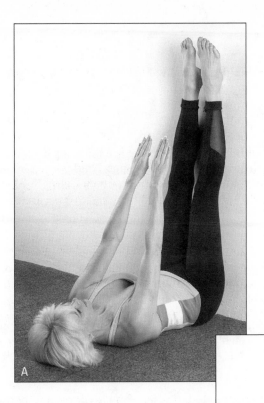

Figure 15-4:
Keep your
chin up
during the
Wall Reach.

Butterfly Lift

Work your upper abs with this effective exercise.

Getting set

Lie on your back so that the soles of your feet are touching each other. Let your knees fall out to the side like butterfly wings. Hold your chin up and neck straight. Place your arms across your chest (see Figure 15-5A).

The exercise

Squeeze or contract your upper abdominals to lift your upper torso off the floor (see Figure 15-5B). Slowly return to start. Do five to ten repetitions. As you progress, work up to 10 to 20 repetitions.

Don't be as concerned about the height of the lift as you are about using correct form. A lift of little height done with good technique is far more effective than a sloppy move that has reached a higher distance. Sometimes less is more.

Exhale during the point of exertion or when you lift your upper body up. Inhale as you return to start.

Other options

Extend your arms: Extending your arms between your legs makes this exercise easier. Be patient with yourself until your abs get stronger.

Place your hands behind your head: Do this for a greater challenge. Do not lace your fingers — rest them behind your ears. Keep your elbows to the side, bent and open.

Adjust your legs and feet: Adjusting your legs and feet to be either closer or farther away from your buttocks creates a better leverage for the move that is best for your body size. Try moving them until you find a comfortable position.

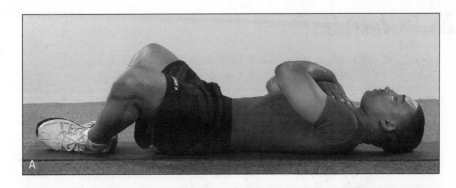

Figure 15-5:
The
Butterfly
Lift tones up
the belly.

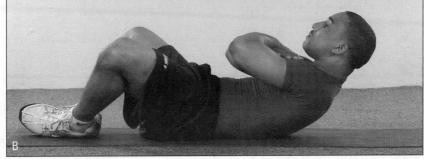

The Chair Lift

The Chair Lift is not a ride up the mountain at a ski resort, but used properly it will take you to the top of your upper abs form.

Getting set

Lie on your back. Raise your legs up and let your calves rest on the seat of a chair for support. Your hips and knees should form a 90-degree angle. Place your hands behind your head with elbows bent and out to the side. Do not lace your fingers, but rest them behind your ears (see Figure 15-6A).

Keep your butt as close to the chair as possible while maintaining a 90-degree angle. The further away you go, the less challenging the exercise.

The exercise

Contract the upper abs to lift your upper body off the floor. Pause and hold the squeeze (see Figure 15-6B). Slowly return to start and immediately repeat the move. Do five to ten repetitions. As you progress, work up to 10 to 20 repetitions.

Don't jerk your head and neck to lift your upper torso up, which could cause injury. The movement should come from the contraction of your upper abs.

Exhale when you lift your upper torso up. Inhale to return to start. (It helps to remember that exhalation occurs during the most difficult part of the move.)

Other options

Adjust your arms: If you are a beginner, you can start by doing the exercise with your arms extended out to your sides. Take it to an intermediate level by crossing your hands over your chest.

Press your feet into a wall: As you become more advanced, you can forget the chair altogether. Maintaining a 90-degree angle, press your feet into a wall as you complete the move.

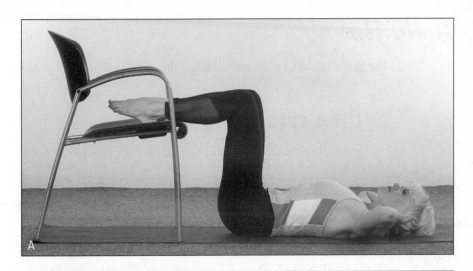

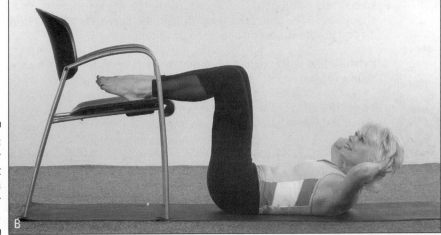

Figure 15-6:
The Chair
Lift
strengthens
the upper
abs.

Belly Up

The Belly Up works your entire midsection with an emphasis on the upper abs.

Getting set

Lie on your back with knees bent and pointed up toward the ceiling. Feet flat on the floor, rest your hands on the top of your thighs. Lift your shoulders off the floor (see Figure 15-7A).

The exercise

Slowly lift your upper body up until your hands just slightly go past your knees. Pause and hold (see Figure 15-7B). Slowly return to start. Briefly let the shoulder blades touch the floor. Repeat the move. Do five to ten repetitions. As you progress, work up to 10 to 20 repetitions.

Exhale when you contract your abs to lift your upper body. Inhale on the return to start.

To get the most benefit out of this exercise, it is critical that you hold your abs in tight throughout the entire move.

Other options

Draft a friend: If the Belly Up is too much of a challenge, draft a friend into helping you. He or she can assist you by holding down your feet until you are stronger. If no one is available, you can secure your feet under a sofa or a bed.

Slow down the count: Slowing down the count will increase the difficulty of this exercise. Try lifting and lowering for a count of four rather than two. Maintain correct form throughout.

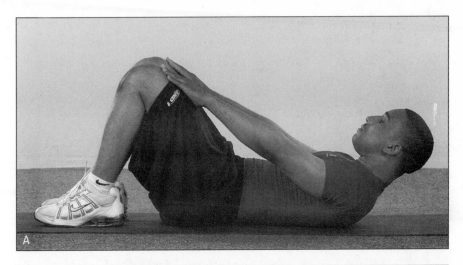

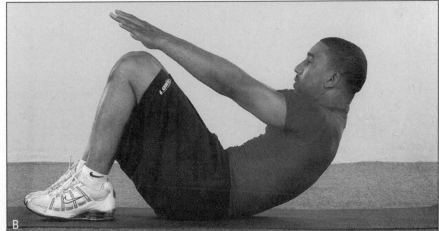

Figure 15-7:
This move
takes your
upper abs
belly up.

Chapter 16

Back to the Future: Lower Back

Strengthening your lower back for the future is something you shouldn't turn your back on. After all, the lower back is responsible for two major functions: It helps you bend backwards, and it maintains a stable position when you move another part of your body.

If you have weak lower back muscles, an action as simple as sitting in a movie theatre or in front of your computer suddenly seems like a monumental task. The stress on your spine is compounded by sitting with slouched or sloppy posture. Certainly, it helps to avoid sitting for too long by taking frequent breaks. Doing the exercises in this chapter can build lower back strength and flexibility that can last a lifetime.

Many people with lower back problems are quick to do abdominal exercises to help relieve the pain. This is a very wise choice, but it's not the entire answer. To help alleviate lower back pain and prevent injury, you need to work the part of your body fitness experts refer to as the *core*. The core muscles consist of the lower back muscles as well as the abdominals. If one group is stronger than the other, balance is lost, posture is off, and you're likely to start feeling back pain. It's the union of a strong lower back and abdominal muscles that leads to a healthy core. (For more information on the core and how working it can strengthen your lower back, visit Chapters 13 through 15.)

If a healthy strong back isn't enough to motivate you to master these moves, how about a leaner look? A strong, healthy lower back lends itself to better posture, and better posture promotes a standing tall attitude: We all look thinner and better when we stand or sit tall. It takes strong lower back muscles to achieve this appealing stance. So get started on your way to healthier back by using the exercises in this chapter.

Getting to Know Your Lower Back

Understanding basic anatomy of the lower back can help you center in on the exact area you are working on. (Refer to Chapter 1 for more on how creating a mental and physical plan can affect your lower back results.) The lower back muscle group you should know about is called the *erector spinae.* I wish I had some cute slang name to give you for this powerful muscle group, but I'm afraid I don't, so you can simply call it the **lower back.** If you touch yourself on each side of your spine just above your hips, you can feel the bottom part of the erector spinae (see Figure 16-1). It runs along your lower spine. Whether your lower back is bending back or remaining stable, the erector spinae works in conjunction with your abdominal muscles.

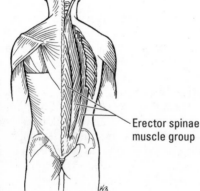

Figure 16-1: The powerful lower back muscle group.

Erector spinae muscle group

Lower Back Exercise Techniques

Use the following lower back hints to enhance your workout:

✔ **Listen to your body:** Because the lower back is such a sensitive area, you must listen to your body. If you currently have back troubles, are prone to injury, or are experiencing any pain during the exercises, please consult with your physician. (Also refer to Chapter 1 for more on medical, health, and safety issues.)

✔ **Warm-up and stretch:** Always do an aerobic warm-up before your lower back routine and make sure that you stretch at the end of the routine. Try the stretching moves found in Chapter 4.

✔ **Get the right equipment:** A lower back routine requires minimal equipment. All you need is a fitness mat, rug, or towel. No more excuses!

✔ **Breathe properly:** Be sure to exhale during exertion, which is the most difficult part of the exercise, and whatever you do, don't hold your breath.

✔ **Don't jerk:** In order for lower back exercises to be successful, you must use slow, controlled movements. Jerky form creates too much stress on the back.

✔ **Use your legs and buns:** When lifting, you should bend and use your legs and buns to assist you with the movement.

✔ **Arch your back slightly:** When doing lower back extension exercises, arch your back only slightly. It helps if you think of elongating or lengthening the spine rather than raising the lower back up high.

Dead Lift with Bent Knee

This powerful move works to strengthen the lower back as well as the hamstrings and glutes. Try doing it the next time you take a break from the computer or during a commercial while you're watching TV.

Getting set

Start by standing with your feet flat on the floor shoulder-width apart.

Be aware of your posture. Straighten out your spine so that it remains in neutral alignment (see Figure 16-2A). That just means the vertebrae are held up in a straight line, one on top of each other (more on this in Chapter 1).

The exercise

With your back straight, flex, or in other words bend, from your hips and reach down till your hands hit just below your knees. Your knees should be slightly bent (see Figure 16-2B). Using your legs and lower back to push off, slowly return to the starting position. Keep your head up throughout this entire exercise in a neutral position. If you are a beginner, do five or fewer repetitions. As you progress, gradually work up to 15 repetitions.

Other options

Use weights: To make this move more advanced, do it with a weight in each hand. As your lower back becomes stronger, you can increase the resistance. (For more information, on how to increase weight safely, review Chapter 3.)

Pause the movement: Take this move to an intermediate level by pausing at the bent forward position. Hold for a slow count of four before returning to start.

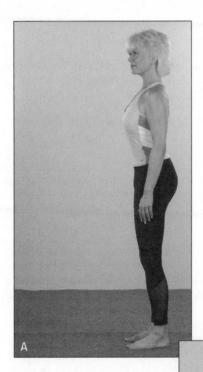

Figure 16-2:
Do the Dead
Lift with
Bent Knee
during
commer-
cials.

Pelvic Tilt

The Pelvic Tilt uses the lower spine to strengthen lower back stability. It's a tiny move that works the abdominals and hamstrings in its action.

Getting set

Lie on the floor on your back with your arms behind your head. Bend your knees so that your feet are flat on the floor about hip-width apart. Contract or squeeze your abdominals as you press your back down (see Figure 16-3A).

The exercise

Hold your back on the floor as you tilt your hips to raise your butt about an inch off the floor — 2 inches maximum. Stay in this position for a moment (see Figure 16-3B).

Slowly bring your butt back to start. As a beginner, you can do five or fewer repetitions. Gradually increase up to 20 or even more repetitions.

You may want to lift the lower back up. For the Pelvic Tilt to be effective, keep the lower back in neutral alignment for the duration of the exercise. Do not raise your head, neck, or shoulders. Remember not to arch your back.

Other options

Use a chair: To make the pelvic tilt easier, do it with your feet placed up on a chair. Bend your knees in a 90-degree angle so that your upper legs are perpendicular to the floor.

Raise your hips: Make the move more difficult by starting it with hands on your hips. (Refer to the Lower Back Lift exercise next up in this chapter for a more detailed description of how to do the move.)

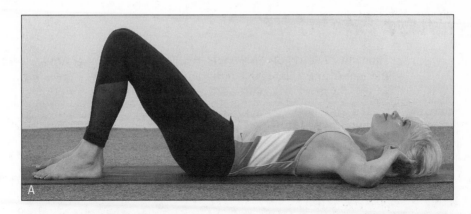

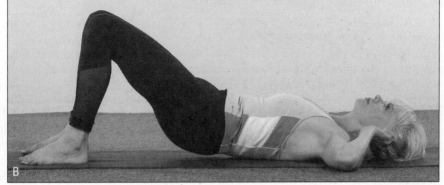

Figure 16-3:
Don't lift
your pelvis
higher than
2 inches.

Lower Back Lift

The Lower Back Lift is an advanced move that strengthens the lower back and actively stimulates the glutes and hamstrings. If you are a beginner, first perfect the Pelvic Tilt exercise, described earlier.

Getting set

Lie on the floor on your back. Bend your knees so that your feet are flat on the ground shoulder-width apart. Your hands should be resting on your hips (see Figure 16-4A).

The exercise

Squeeze your butt and lower back muscles as you lift your hips off the floor to a raised position (see Figure 16-4B).

Your shoulders, upper back, and feet are the only parts that should have any contact with the floor. Do not let your butt sag and do not arch your back. It is best to keep your spine in neutral alignment (see Chapter 1).

From the raised position, lift your hips another 5 inches without arching your back. (See Figure 16-4C.) Pause for a few seconds and slowly return to the first raised position (not the floor). When beginning this challenge, repeat the move five times. As you progress gradually, work up to 20 repetitions.

Other options

Make it easier: Take this move to a slightly easier level. Rather than raising your lower back up to the second raised position, stop at the first lift. Pause at the first lift and then slowly return to the floor to start.

Make it more advanced: Dare to advance this exercise by holding for a count of four in the second raised position. It helps to hold your abdominals in tight and to squeeze your butt and lower back.

Lift one leg: For an even greater challenge, extend one leg out completely or keep that foot off the ground with the bent knee position.

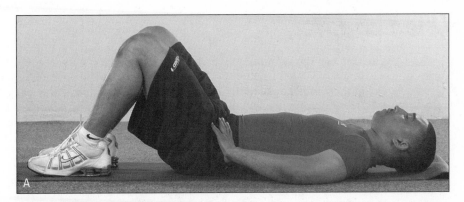

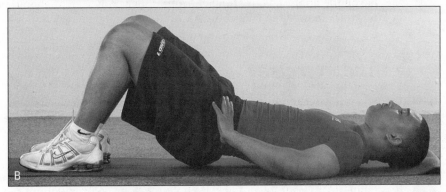

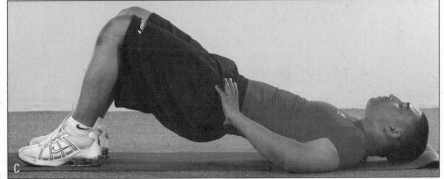

Figure 16-4:
This move
isolates the
lower back
muscles.

One Leg Lift

The One Leg Lift emphasizes the lower back muscles.

Doing this move consistently may help to alleviate some lower back discomfort. However, you should use caution. Whenever you experience a sharp pain in this or any lower back exercise, consult with your physician.

Getting set

Lie on the floor on your stomach. Your upper body weight should be resting on your elbows (see Figure 16-5A).

The exercise

Squeeze your buns and the back of your legs as you lift one leg up (see Figure 16-5B). Pause for a second and return to start. Repeat the move ten times on each leg.

It is critical that you do not lift the leg up higher than what is comfortable. In fact, the height of the lift is not nearly as important as the gentle contraction (squeeze) of your lower back. Do not arch your back, and don't swing your legs up and down. Keep the movement simple and small. Hold your abdominals in tight to support your back.

Other options

Kneel: This is a great beginner, lower back exercise. Kneel on all fours, and then lift and extend one leg out directly behind you. This puts very little stress on the lower spine.

Use ankle weights: If you have accomplished the One Leg Lift, try doing it with ankle weights. Use only the amount of weight you can handle without losing the correct form. (Refer to Chapter 3 for tips on how to increase weight safely.)

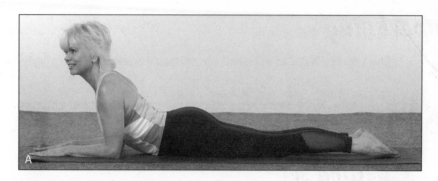

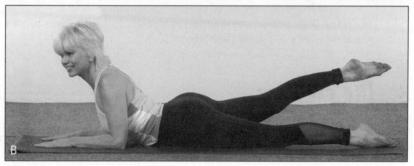

Figure 16-5:
The One
Leg Lift
strengthens
the lower
back.

Superbeing

The Superbeing is an excellent lower back exercise. Do it regularly for strong results.

If you experience pain during this or any exercise or have a history of lower back problems, consult with your physician.

Getting set

Lie on the floor in a prone position (on your stomach). Your arms should be extended over your head (see Figure 16-6A).

The exercise

Lift your upper body off the floor at the same time you lift your legs up (see Figure 16-6B). Pause and hold for a slow count of four. Return to start. Repeat the move five times.

Lift the arms and legs up only as high as is comfortable. You should feel a gentle contraction or squeeze in the lower back rather than excessive pressure on the spine.

Hold your abdominal muscles in tight. Squeeze your butt and the back of your legs to help facilitate the movement.

Other options

Place your arms at the side: Doing the move with your arms down at your side is easier.

Place your hands behind your head: Placing your hands behind your head is more difficult.

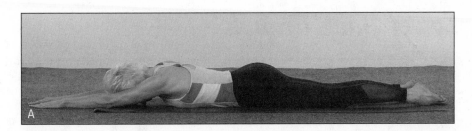

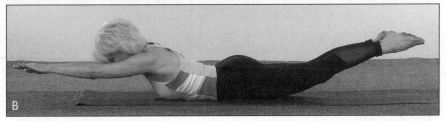

Figure 16-6:
Lift up only
as high as is
comfortable.

Lower Back Crunch

This move is the exact opposite of an abs crunch. An abs crunch works the abdominals, whereas a Lower Back Crunch works just what the name says — the lower back. Together, the abdominals and the lower back make up the *core* of your body. You need exercises from both muscle groups to balance your body. The Lower Back Crunch is a perfect compliment to your core routine. (For more core information and some effective abdominal exercises, see Chapters 13 through 15.)

Getting set

Lie on the floor in a prone position (on your stomach). Your hands should be behind your head (see Figure 16-7A).

The exercise

Squeeze your butt and lower back muscles as you lift your upper torso approximately 3 to 5 inches from the floor. Pause and hold for a few seconds (see Figure 16-7B). Slowly return to start. Repeat five times. As you progress, work up to ten repetitions.

Other options

Hold your feet down: To simplify the move, have a partner hold your ankles for added support.

Place your arms at your sides: To decrease the level of difficulty, place your arms at your sides.

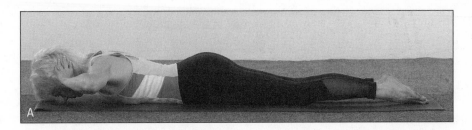

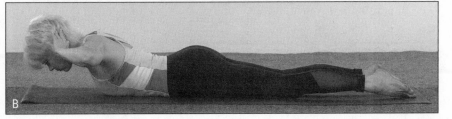

Figure 16-7:
This
movement
builds core
strength.

Part V

Customizing Your Workouts and Maximizing Your Results

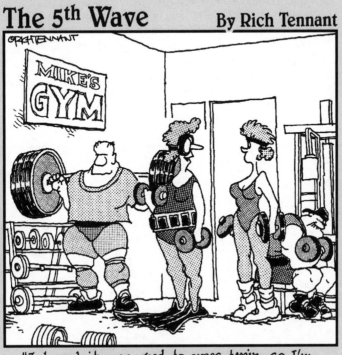

The 5th Wave   By Rich Tennant

MIKE'S GYM

"I heard it was good to cross-train, so I'm mixing my weight training with scuba diving."

In this part . . .

1 provide several fun, fast-fitness and full-course fitness menus that are a challenging 10 minutes each as well as 20 minutes or more, so you can achieve quicker results. But you also need to know how you can eat lots of wonderful foods and still look great without going on some crazy diet. So I explain in simple terms the necessary nutrients your body needs and show you how to keep a food journal to record your progress and keep you going in the right direction. I also outline the many benefits to adding a cardiovascular workout to your program. If you travel a lot you can still take fitness on the road. I offer lots of tips to help you not only reach your immediate goals but take them beyond.

Chapter 17

Fast-Fitness Menus to Go: Ten Minutes Each

In This Chapter

▶ Customizing the menus to meet your needs
▶ Getting the most out of the menus
▶ Picking personal fast-fitness menus

*I*magine this scenario. You look in the mirror at your rear end and think "Whopper." You can't see your feet due to a belly you call "Big Mac." Your confidence may be sinking like a "Sub," and your chin says "Double, Double." From now on, rather than over-ordering from the drive-thru fast-food menu, try one of my fast-fitness menus. In this chapter, you take control with personalized, self-service, fast-fitness choices. Choose from several ten minute tone-up menus, including lean legs, fab abs, buns that cook and more. Instead of fatty fried wings, you can choose arms that are trim and toned. There's even a menu of moves that you can do anytime and anywhere. Order quick results today. Would you like great thighs with that?

Mixing the Menus: Have It Your Way

This chapter has all the menus you need to fill up on fast-fitness success. But, it's up to you to scan the choices and "have it your way." You can interactively mix the menus and the exercises to create a personal plan that works for you. The options are endless. You can also come up with your own. Using the following tips, create versatile, personal plans that fit your lifestyle and change as them to.

✔ **Use each menu on its own:** You can make an excellent choice just by using each menu as it appears in this chapter. I've placed the exercises in an effective order. The menus are simple to follow, and they really do work!

✔ **Choose different menus on different days:** You may choose to switch your fitness menu plan throughout the week. For example, on day one you can use the Hot Buns menu; day three, Fab Abs; and if you're traveling on day five, Anytime-Anywhere moves. Make it work for you.

✔ **Alternate the menus:** Take advantage of the days between your primary workout. For example, if you want to focus on your legs, you can follow the Lean Legs menu for day one, day three, and day five. However, you can also include the fab abs menu on days two and four, or work out with any of the other menus on alternate days. As long as you don't work the same body part two days in a row, you can maximize the benefits.

✔ **Vary the exercises:** The menus provide a self-contained workout program so you can achieve your desired goals. However, for variety, you can also switch the exercises around with other appropriate moves. I've conveniently placed the chapter numbers next to each exercise. You can use that information to check your form and technique, or substitute the move for another effective one from the corresponding chapter. You've got choices.

✔ **Use the other options:** Each exercise cross-references to the chapter where it's located. Use that helpful information to review the technique, tips, and breathing for each exercise, plus you can use the "Other options" section in this chapter to help you meet your individual needs. You can use the exercise modifications to adjust the exercise to your level of difficulty or just for variety.

Making the Most of Ten Minute Tone-Ups

Before you find and personalize a workout for yourself, follow these guidelines to get the most effective workout and the best results:

✔ Always include an aerobic warm-up before you do your tone-ups for a minimum of five to ten minutes (see Chapter 20 for cardio suggestions) and do stretching at the end of the workout (see Chapter 4).

✔ For maximum results include a full cardiovascular workout daily or at least do cardio on days between your tone-up days. (See Chapter 20.)

✔ Use appropriate weight (see Chapter 3).

✔ Maintain a sensible diet (see Chapter 19).

Selecting a Fun, Fast-Fitness Menu

I've listed all of my fun, fast-fitness menus in this chapter. Each of them can be done in ten minutes and, aside from the Anytime-Anywhere Moves and Fast Circuit Toning, each menu has separate beginner and advanced menus. (Also see the full-course fitness menus in Chapter 18.)

Photocopy or re-create on your computer the cheat sheet in the beginning of the book so you can follow your progress. Simply mark the date at the top of the chart, fill in the exercises for each day using one of the fitness menus in this chapter, and record your repetitions and sets. You can even log your own personal notes, such as how you feel during a session, moves you need to work on, moves you've gotten better at, or the names of guests you forgot to invite to your upcoming wedding.

Don't get frustrated if you see an exercise and can't remember which one it is — just check out the chapter number to the right of the move and flip there for a quick refresher as well as variations of the original exercise that tailor the move to your fitness level.

Toning up your total body

If you have only 30 days and need a complete overhaul or want to shed a few inches, this menu is for you. Well, okay — you may not be able to achieve an Adonis or Venus physique overnight, but toning up totally is very realistic. If you're a beginner, head to the menu in Table 17-1; if you're advanced, check out Table 17-2.

Table 17-1	***Fast-Fitness Total Body Beginner Menu**	
Day 1	*Day 3*	*Day 5*
Wall Push-ups (Chapter 5)	Squats (Chapter 11)	Lift and Cross (Chapter 13)
Modified Push-ups (Chapter 5)	Standing Heel Curl (Chapter 10)	Lower Abs Lift (Chapter 14)
One Arm Dumbbell Row (Chapter 6)	Standing Calf (Chapter 12)	Pelvic Tilt (Chapter 16)
Upright Row (Chapter 7)	Legs Apart Thigh Flexion (Chapter 9)	Seated Same Time Biceps Curl (Chapter 8)
External & Internal Rotation (Chapter 7)	Standing Hip Abduction w/ Band (Chapter 9)	Over the Head Triceps Extension (Chapter 8)

*Do an aerobic warm-up and end with a stretch. On days in between your tone-ups, do cardio. Eat sensibly.

Table 17-2	*Fast-Fitness Total Body Advanced Menu	
Day 1	**Day 3**	**Day 5**
Flat Bench Press (Chapter 5)	Lunge (Chapter 10)	Crossed Leg Side Crunch (Chapter 13)
Incline Fly (Chapter 5)	Standing Hip Abduction w/ Band (Chapter 9)	Tummy Pull Leg Push (Chapter 14)
Seated Rear Deltoid Lift (Chapter 7)	Legs Apart Thigh Flexion (Chapter 9)	Lower Back Crunch (Chapter 16)
Kneeling 2 Arm Row (Chapter 6)	Resistance Band Squat (Chapter 10)	Lying Triceps Extension (Chapter 8)
External & Internal Rotation (Chapter 7)	Great Legs Band Stretch (Chapter 10)	Seated Concentration Biceps Curl (Chapter 8)

Do an aerobic warm-up and end with a stretch. On days in between your tone-ups, do cardio. Eat sensibly.

Shaping your chest, upper back and shoulders

This menu can cut your upper torso into a shape that commands attention. With the right discipline, you can sculpt your upper back, chest, and shoulders. Beginners use Table 17-3; if you're advanced, use Table 17-4.

Table 17-3	*Fast-Fitness Upper Body Beginner Menu	
Day 1	**Day 3**	**Day 5**
Isometric Chest Press (Chapter 5)	Wall Push-ups (Chapter 5)	Modified Push-up (Chapter 5)
Upper Back Shoulder Shrug (Chapter 6)	Modified Push-ups (Chapter 5)	Seated Dumbbell Row (Chapter 6)
Bent Forward Row (Chapter 6)	One Arm Dumbbell Row (Chapter 6)	External & Internal Rotations (Chapter 7)
External & Internal Rotations (Chapter 7)	External & Internal Rotations (Chapter 7)	Side Lateral Raise (Chapter 7)
Side Lateral Raise (Chapter 7)	Deltoid Press (Chapter 7)	Upright Row (Chapter 7)

Do an aerobic warm-up and end with a stretch. On days in between your tone-ups, do cardio. Eat sensibly.

Table 17-4	*Fast-Fitness Upper Body Advanced Menu	
Day 1	*Day 3*	*Day 5*
Flat Bench Press (Chapter 5)	Incline Fly (Chapter 5)	Modified Push-up (Chapter 5)
Incline Fly (Chapter 5)	Kneeling Two Arm Row (Chapter 6)	Dumbbell Pullover (Chapter 5)
Bent Forward Row (Chapter 6)	External & Internal Rotations (Chapter 7)	Resistance Band Lat Pulldown (Chapter 6)
External & Internal Rotations (Chapter 7)	Seated Rear Deltoid Lift (Chapter 7)	External & Internal Rotations (Chapter 7)
Deltoid Press (Chapter 7)	Dumbbell Pullover (Chapter 5)	Alternating Lateral Raise (Chapter 7)

Do an aerobic warm-up and end with a stretch. On days in between your tone-ups, do cardio. Eat sensibly.

Getting lean legs now

Get great gams with this fitness menu. Stay true to this menu and walk away with firm thighs, quads, and calves. Beginners use Table 17-5; if you're advanced, check out Table 17-6.

Table 17-5	*Fast-Fitness Lean Legs Beginner Menu	
Day 1	*Day 3*	*Day 5*
Lunge (Chapter 10)	Resistance Band Squat (Chapter 10)	Lunge (Chapter 10)
Outer Thigh Leg Lift (Chapter 9)	Legs Apart Thigh Flexion (Chapter 9)	Standing Hip Abduction w/ Band (Chapter 9)
Inner Thigh Leg Lift (Chapter 9)	Inner Thigh Scissor Cut (Chapter 9)	Legs Apart Thigh Flexion (Chapter 9)
Standing Heel Curl (Chapter 10)	Hamstrings Curl (Chapter 10)	Hamstrings Curl (Chapter 10)
Standing Calf (Chapter 12)	Lifting Calf — Seated (Chapter 12)	Sitting Calf Strengthener (Chapter 12)

Do an aerobic warm-up and end with a stretch. On days in between your tone-ups, do cardio. Eat sensibly.

Table 17-6	*Fast-Fitness Lean Legs Advanced Menu	
Day 1	**Day 3**	**Day 5**
Resistance Band Squat (Chapter 10)	Lunge (Chapter 10)	Great Legs Band Stretch (Chapter 10)
Standing Hip Abduction w/ Band (Chapter 9)	Outer Thigh Leg Lift (Chapter 9)	Legs Apart Thigh Flexion (Chapter 9)
Legs Apart Thigh Flexion (Chapter 9)	Inner Thigh Scissor Cut (Chapter 9)	Standing Hip Abduction w/ Band (Chapter 9)
Standing Heel Curl (Chapter 10)	Hamstrings on a Bench (Chapter 10)	Hamstrings Curl (Chapter 10)
Standing Calf w/ Barbell (Chapter 12)	Raising One Leg Calf Lift (Chapter 12)	Standing Calf w/ Barbell (Chapter 12)

*Do an aerobic warm-up and end with a stretch. On days in between your tone-ups, do cardio. Eat sensibly.

Finding your fab abs and lower back

This menu gets to the core. Follow it strictly and you can see a toned-up difference in 30 days. The secret is to follow the exercise descriptions and techniques that I have described. Concentrate on proper breathing — always exhale on exertion. Besides a great-looking stomach, expect a stronger back and improved stability. Beginners, try Table 17-7; if you're advanced, stick with Table 17-8.

Table 17-7	*Fast-Fitness Fab Abs Beginner Menu	
Day 1	**Day 3**	**Day 5**
Oblique Crunch (Chapter 13)	Lift and Cross (Chapter 13)	Side Waist Toner (Chapter 13)
Lift and Cross (Chapter 13)	Legs Up Lower Abs Lift (Chapter 14)	Seated Leg Lift (Chapter 14)
Lower Abs Lift (Chapter 14)	Seated Leg Lift (Chapter 14)	Wall Reach (Chapter 15)
Crunch (Chapter 15)	Chair Lift (Chapter 15)	Chair Lift (Chapter 15)
Pelvic Tilt (Chapter 16)	Dead Lift w/ Bent Knee (Chapter 16)	Lower Back Lift (Chapter 16)

*Do an aerobic warm-up and end with a stretch. On days in between your tone-ups, do cardio. Eat sensibly.

Table 17-8	*Fast-Fitness Fab Abs Advanced Menu	
Day 1	*Day 3*	*Day 5*
Side Twist (Chapter 13)	Elbow to Knee (Chapter 13)	Crossed Leg Side Crunch (Chapter 13)
Crossed Leg Side Crunch (Chapter 13)	Tummy Pull Leg Push (Chapter 14)	Bicycle (Chapter 14)
Belly Be My Best (Chapter 14)	Bicycle (Chapter 14)	Belly Up (Chapter 15)
Toe Reach (Chapter 15)	Butterfly Lift (Chapter 15)	Toe Reach (Chapter 15)
One Leg Lift (Chapter 16)	Superbeing (Chapter 16)	Lower Back Crunch (Chapter 16)

*Do an aerobic warm-up and end with a stretch. On days in between your tone-ups, do cardio. Eat sensibly.

Cooking up some hot buns

Improve your assets with this menu. These simple yet intense exercises get bottom-line results. Beginners should use Table 17-9, and if you're advanced, you should use Table 17-10.

Table 17-9	*Fast-Fitness Hot Buns Beginner Menu	
Day 1	*Day 3*	*Day 5*
Lunge (Chapter 10)	Lunge (Chapter 10)	Lunge (Chapter 10)
Squats (Chapter 11)	Bottoms Up Butt Lift (Chapter 11)	Squats (Chapter 11)
Anytime Standing Bun Burner (Chapter 11)	Great Legs Band Stretch (Chapter 10)	Resistance Band Squat (Chapter 10)
Floor Butt Lift (Chapter 11)	Floor Butt Lift (Chapter 11)	Anytime Standing Bun Burner (Chapter 11)
Bottoms Up Butt Lift (Chapter 11)	Squats (Chapter 11)	Floor Butt Lift (Chapter 11)

*Do an aerobic warm-up and end with a stretch. On days in between your tone-ups, do cardio. Eat sensibly.

Table 17-10	*Fast-Fitness Hot Buns Advanced Menu	
Day 1	*Day 3*	*Day 5*
Squats (Chapter 11)	Lunge (Chapter 10)	Kick Butt (Chapter 11)
Floor Butt Lift (Chapter 11)	Bun Blast Off (Chapter 11)	Great Legs Band Stretch (Chapter 10)
Great Legs Band Stretch (Chapter 10)	Resistance Band Squat (Chapter 10)	Floor Butt Lift (Chapter 11)
Kick Butt (Chapter 11)	Kick Butt (Chapter 11)	Bottoms Up Butt Lift (Chapter 11)
Bun Blast Off (Chapter 11)	Bottoms Up Butt Lift (Chapter 11)	Bun Blast Off (Chapter 11)

Do an aerobic warm-up and end with a stretch. On days in between your tone-ups, do cardio. Eat sensibly.

Toning your arms

Flabby arms can make you seem heavier and even older than you really are. However in 30 days, you can have firm results in hand if you stick to the plan. Beginners, use Table 17-11; if you're advanced, use Table 17-12.

Table 17-11	*Fast-Fitness Toning Your Arms Beginner Menu	
Day 1	*Day 3*	*Day 5*
Seated Same Time Biceps Curl (Chapter 8)	Seated Same Time Biceps Curl (Chapter 8)	Seated Same Time Biceps Curl (Chapter 8)
Angled Same Time Biceps Curl (Chapter 8)	Seated Concentration Biceps Curl (Chapter 8)	Angled Same Time Biceps Curl (Chapter 8)
Over the Head Triceps Extension (Chapter 8)	Lying Triceps Extension (Chapter 8)	Over the Head Triceps Extension (Chapter 8)
Triceps Dip (Chapter 8)	Triceps Dip (Chapter 8)	One Sided Triceps Kickback (Chapter 8)
Wrist & Reverse Wrist Curl (Chapter 8)	Wrist & Reverse Wrist Curl (Chapter 8)	Wrist & Reverse Wrist Curl (Chapter 8)

Do an aerobic warm-up and end with a stretch. On days in between your tone-ups, do cardio. Eat sensibly.

Table 17-12	*Fast-Fitness Toning Your Arms Advanced Menu	
Day 1	*Day 3*	*Day 5*
Seated Same Time Biceps Curl (Chapter 8)	Seated Concentration Biceps Curl (Chapter 8)	Seated Same Time Biceps Curl (Chapter 8)
Angled Same Time Biceps Curl (Chapter 8)	Angled Same Time Biceps Curl (Chapter 8)	Seated Concentration Biceps Curl (Chapter 8)
Triceps Dip (Chapter 8)	One Sided Triceps Kickback (Chapter 8)	Lying Triceps Extension (Chapter 8)
Lying Triceps Extension (Chapter 8)	Over the Head Triceps Extension (Chapter 8)	One Sided Triceps Kickback (Chapter 8)
Wrist & Reverse Wrist Curl (Chapter 8)	Wrist & Reverse Wrist Curl (Chapter 8)	Wrist & Reverse Wrist Curl (Chapter 8)

Do an aerobic warm-up and end with a stretch. On days in between your tone-ups, do cardio. Eat sensibly.

Firming up with fast circuit toning

To experience circuit toning, you simply perform a series of exercises quickly, one after the other without a rest between them. Bear in mind that I said *quickly* and not *sloppily*. Correct form must always come first. In addition to the tone-up benefits of the exercises in this menu, your heart and lungs get a great workout, too. However, on days between your fast circuit toning, include an aerobic activity and always eat a sensible diet (see Chapter 20 for cardio-vascular choices and Chapter 19 for diet information).

In Table 17-13, I've pre-packaged a fast *circuit toning* program that works the whole body. Regardless of your fitness level, you can use the following menu. You can tailor it to your fitness need by the number of repetitions and sets that you perform. In general, beginners should do five repetitions of one or two circuit toning sets. Advanced exercises should do ten repetitions of two or three circuit toning sets. In addition, like all the menus in this chapter, you can also use another option of the exercise to make it easier or more difficult — just check out the chapter reference next to each exercise in the menu.

You should use about 15 to 20 percent less weight than you normally would for the exercises that require dumbbells, to compensate for the rapid movements.

Resting results

To achieve fast results, take a rest! Never do the same muscle group two days in a row. This allows for your muscles to recover from the work that they have done. In fact, it is actually in the recovery that the tone up occurs. Resting in between sets while doing your menus can also make a difference. The longer you rest between exercises, the more weight or resistance you can handle. Body builders usually rest one minute or longer. They need a longer rest because they are lifting excessive weights. In general though, 30 seconds of rest is enough time between sets for safe, quick tone-up results. Resting for two weeks between sets is not effective.

Table 17-13	*Fast Circuit Toning All Levels Menu	
Day 1 (Chest, Shoulders, and Upper Back)	*Day 3 (Buns and Legs)*	*Day 5 (Arms and Abs)*
Shadow Box (30 sec.)	Run in Place (30 sec.)	Jump Rope (30 sec.)
Flat Bench Press (Chapter 5)	Lunge (Chapter 10)	Seated Same Time Biceps Curl (Chapter 8)
Bent Forward Row (Chapter 6)	Hamstrings Curl (Chapter 10)	Over the Head Triceps Extension (Chapter 8)
Shadow Box (30 sec.)	Run in Place (30 sec.)	Jump Rope (30 sec.)
Deltoid Press (Chapter 7)	Resistance Band Squat (Chapter 10)	Oblique Crunch (Chapter 13)
Dumbbell Pullover (Chapter 5)	Inner & Outer Thigh Leg Lift (Chapter 9)	One Leg Lift (Chapter 16)

Do an aerobic warm-up and end with a stretch. On days in between your tone-ups, do cardio. Eat sensibly.

Getting pumped anytime, anywhere

Do the menu in Table 17-14 everywhere. Incorporate these simple exercises into your life for long-lasting, quick tone-up results. Do the toning-up moves on the left side of the page to strengthen and tone up your muscles. The rejuvenating moves (stretches, actually) on the right side of the page can improve flexibility, and they just plain feel great! Plus, with 30 days to reach your goals, all of these Anytime-Anywhere moves matter.

Table 17-14	***Anytime-Anywhere All Levels Menu**
Toning-up Moves	_Rejuvenating Moves_
Isometric Chest Press (Chapter 5)	Neck Stretch (Chapter 4)
Wall Push-ups (Chapter 5)	Shoulder Rolls (Chapter 4)
Upper Back Shoulder Shrug (Chapter 6)	Upward, Backward, and Forward Reach (Chapter 4)
Deltoid Press (Chapter 7)	Quadriceps Stretch (Chapter 4)
Seated Same Time Biceps Curl (Chapter 8)	Calf Stretch (Chapter 4)
Triceps Dip (Chapter 8)	Standing Abs (Chapter 4)
Lunge (Chapter10)	
Squats (Chapter 11)	
Standing Heel Curl (Chapter 10)	
Anytime Standing Saddlebag Toner (Chapter 9)	
Anytime Standing Bun Burner (Chapter 11)	
Standing Calf (Chapter 12)	
Seated Leg Lift (Chapter 14)	
Dead Lift w/ Bent Knee (Chapter 16)	

*Do an aerobic warm-up and end with a stretch. On days in between your tone-ups, do cardio. Eat sensibly.

Chapter 18

Full-Course Fitness Menus: 20 Minutes or More

....

In This Chapter

▶ Personalizing the menus to reach your goals

▶ Getting tips for the best results

▶ Selecting full-course fitness menus

....

*F*ast food and fast fitness may be fine during a hectic day. However, how sad it is to go through life without savoring the palatable pleasures of fine dining and full-course fitness. In this chapter, I provide a sumptuous banquet of full-course fitness menus. Devour the information to your heart's content. Spending 20 minutes or more on a fitness feast can actually help you achieve your tone-up goals even faster. Begin with an aerobic warm-up appetizer and then select an entrée from one of the full-course fitness menus. Incorporate these menus into a delicious lifetime of health and wellness.

Mixing the Menus

This chapter has plenty of full-course fitness menus to wet your appetite. Use them in countless ways for a 20-minute or more workout. You play a proactive part in mixing and matching them to form your own personal plan that's right for you and your lifestyle — bon appetit!

✔ **Use each menu solo:** You can use each full-course fitness menu on its own. Because they're all-inclusive, you don't have to waste any of your valuable time sorting out exercises. The menus are simple to follow and effective. Just pick a plan and do it.

✔ **Use different menus on different days:** For variety, you may select a different menu on different days. This can prove to be beneficial because a wider range of muscle parts are activated. For example, on Day 1, you can do the Shaping Your Abs and Lower Back menu; Day 3, Firming Your Fanny; and Day 5, Full-Course Circuit Toning. In one week, you can target every major muscle group. Customize the menus to meet your needs.

✔ **Use different menus on alternate days:** Since you probably don't think twice about eating everyday, why should you think twice about including a full-course fitness menu on the days in between your primary workout? For example, if your target is Lean Legs and Gams, you can do that menu on Days 1, 3, and 5. On Days 2 and 4, you could use the Defining Your Arms menu for a total appendage advantage. As long as you don't work the same body part two days in a row, you can reap full-course fitness benefits. If 20 minutes can't be spared, opt for a fast-fitness menu on alternate days (see Chapter 17).

✔ **Vary the exercises:** You can achieve your fitness goals with these prepackaged menus. However, it's fun to cultivate a taste for other movements. Feel free to switch the exercises around with other appropriate moves. Just follow the chapter numbers next to each exercise to find substitutes to the prepackaged menu moves; use those chapter references to also check your form and technique.

✔ **Check the other options:** Each exercise cross-references to the chapter where it's located. In addition to reviewing the techniques, tips, and other good stuff, remember to check out the "Other options" component of each exercise. The modifications offered can personalize your plan to the utmost degree. Now, not only the menus but each specific exercise can be adjusted to your individual level of difficulty.

✔ **Increase cardio minutes:** No full-course fitness menu is complete without a 20-minute or more cardiovascular workout. Do a full aerobic activity two or three times a week. Dine on cardio to your heart's content.

Getting Tips for the Best Workout Results

Although each menu gives you all you need, following these guidelines gets you on your way to the most effective workout and the best results:

✔ On days between your workouts, include an aerobic activity for a minimum of 20 to 30 minutes (see Chapter 20 for other cardiovascular choices).

✔ Always include an aerobic warm-up at the start of your workout and stretch at the end (see Chapter 4).

✔ Use appropriate weight (see Chapter 3).

✔ Maintain a sensible diet (see Chapter 19).

Choosing a Full-Course Fitness Menu

Accept the exciting challenge of taking fast fitness to a full-course level. Each of these menus can be done in 20 minutes or more and comes in a beginner as well as an advanced version. I've prepared them so that they fit neatly into the cheat sheet workout charts in the beginning of the book. Photocopy the cheat sheets or recreate them on your computer to follow your personal progress. Simply write the date at the top of the cheat sheet chart you select (you can select a three-day and a seven-day tone-up chart). Fill in the blanks on the cheat sheet with the name of each exercise from your choice of menus in this chapter or from Chapter 17. You can keep track of your sets and repetitions in the spaces provided. Feel free to scribble notes in the corresponding area or anywhere on the chart. These menus can be adopted to your personal level, are simple to use and can produce a lifetime of health and wellness.

To simplify your program, I've listed the chapter number after each exercise so you can easily flip back and check out the proper technique.

Conditioning your total body

This menu is truly the chef's special. The workout caters to every part of your body. You can tone up your entire physique with these moves. Try to take it beyond your 30-day target date for a lifetime of body-conditioned bliss. Beginners should check out Table 18-1; if you're advanced, check out Table 18-2.

Table 18-1	*Full-Course Fitness Total Body Beginner Menu	
Day 1	*Day 3*	*Day 5*
Isometric Chest Press (Chapter 5)	Lunge (Chapter 10)	Oblique Crunch (Chapter 13)
Wall Push-ups (Chapter 5)	Squats (Chapter 11)	Lower Abs Lift (Chapter 14)
Modified Push-ups (Chapter 5)	Inner Thigh Leg Lift (Chapter 9)	Crunch (Chapter 15)
Seated Dumbbell Row (Chapter 6)	Outer Thigh Leg Lift (Chapter 9)	One Leg Lift (Chapter 16)
Upper Back Shoulder Shrug (Chapter 6)	Floor Butt Lift (Chapter 11)	Seated Same Time Biceps Curl (Chapter 8)

(continued)

Table 18-1 *(continued)*

Day 1	Day 3	Day 5
External & Internal Rotation (Chapter 7)	Bottoms Up Butt Lift (Chapter 11)	Angled Same Time Biceps Curl (Chapter 8)
Upright Row (Chapter 7)	Standing Heel Curl (Chapter 10)	Triceps Dip (Chapter 8)
Side Lateral Raise (Chapter 7)	Raising One Leg Calf Lift (Chapter 12)	Over the Head Triceps Extension (Chapter 8)

*Do an aerobic warm-up and end with a stretch. On days in between your tone-ups, do cardio. Eat sensibly.

Table 18-2   *Full-Course Fitness Total Body Advanced Menu

Day 1	Day 3	Day 5
Flat Bench Press (Chapter 5)	Lunge (Chapter 10)	Side Twist (Chapter 13)
Incline Fly (Chapter 5)	Resistance Band Squat (Chapter 10)	Legs up Lower Abs Lift (Chapter 14)
Dumbbell Pullover (Chapter 5)	Hams on a Bench (Chapter 10)	Belly Up (Chapter 15)
Bent Forward Row (Chapter 6)	Standing Hip Abduction w/Band (Chapter 9)	Lower Back Crunch (Chapter 16)
Kneeling 2 Arm Row (Chapter 6)	Inner Thigh Scissor Cut (Chapter 9)	Seated Concentration Biceps Curl (Chapter 8)
Seated Rear Deltoid Lift (Chapter 7)	Bun Blast off (Chapter 11)	Lying Triceps Extension (Chapter 8)
Alternating Lateral Raise (Chapter 7)	Great Legs Band Stretch (Chapter 10)	One Sided Triceps Kickback (Chapter 8)
External & Internal Rotation (Chapter 7)	Sitting Calf Strengthener (Chapter 12)	Wrist & Reverse Wrist Curls (Chapter 8)

*Do an aerobic warm-up and end with a stretch. On days in between your tone-ups, do cardio. Eat sensibly.

Sculpting your chest, upper back and shoulders

Strengthen and shape your upper torso with this menu. Sculpt your personal best chest, upper back, and shoulders. Dedication to doing these moves can make you stand tall and proud. Beginners should follow Table 18-3, and those of you who are advanced should follow Table 18-4.

Table 18-3	*Full-Course Fitness Chest, Upper Back and Shoulder Sculpting Beginner Menu	
Day 1	*Day 3*	*Day 5*
Isometric Chest Press (Chapter 5)	Isometric Chest Press (Chapter 5)	Modified Push-ups (Chapter 5)
Wall Push-ups (Chapter 5)	Wall Push-ups (Chapter 5)	Flat Bench Press (Chapter 5)
Upper Back Shoulder Shrug (Chapter 6)	Modified Push-ups (Chapter 5)	Seated Dumbbell Row (Chapter 6)
Bent Forward Row (Chapter 6)	One Arm Dumbbell Row (Chapter 6)	One Arm Dumbbell Row (Chapter 6)
Seated Dumbbell Row (Chapter 6)	Resistance Band Lat Pull Down (Chapter 6)	Upper Back Shoulder Shrug (Chapter 6)
External & Internal Rotation (Chapter 7)	External & Internal Rotation (Chapter 7)	External & Internal Rotation (Chapter 7)
Side Lateral Raise (Chapter 7)	Deltoid Press (Chapter 7)	Upright Row (Chapter 7)
Resistance Band Lat Pull Down (Chapter 6)	Side Lateral Raise (Chapter 7)	Deltoid Press (Chapter 7)

Do an aerobic warm-up and end with a stretch. On days in between your tone-ups, do cardio. Eat sensibly.

Table 18-4	*Full-Course Fitness Chest, Upper Back and Shoulder Sculpting Advanced Menu	
Day 1	*Day 3*	*Day 5*
Flat Bench Press (Chapter 5)	Incline Fly (Chapter 5)	Modified Push-ups (Chapter 5)
Incline Fly (Chapter 5)	Flat Bench Press (Chapter 5)	Incline Fly (Chapter 5)
Dumbbell Pullover (Chapter 5)	Modified Push-ups (Chapter 5)	Dumbbell Pullover (Chapter 5)
Kneeling 2 Arm Row (Chapter 6)	Kneeling 2 Arm Row (Chapter 6)	Resistance Band Lat Pull-down (Chapter 6)
Bent Forward Row (Chapter 6)	Resistance Band Lat Pull-down (Chapter 6)	Bent Forward Row (Chapter 6)
External & Internal Rotation (Chapter 7)	External & Internal Rotation (Chapter 7)	Kneeling 2 Arm Row (Chapter 6)
Deltoid Press (Chapter 7)	Seated Rear Deltoid Lift (Chapter 7)	External & Internal Rotation (Chapter 7)
Alternating Lateral Raise (Chapter 7)	Dumbbell Pullover (Chapter 5)	Alternating Lateral Raise (Chapter 7)

Do an aerobic warm-up and end with a stretch. On days in between your tone-ups, do cardio. Eat sensibly.

Looking for some lean legs and gams

Lean and strong legs can be yours with this menu. Do it 3 days a week on alternate days for firm thighs, quads, and calves. Simply spending 20 minutes or more on each session can carry you far into life. If you're a beginner, start with Table 18-5, and then progress to the more advanced menu in Table 18-6 when you're ready.

Table 18-5	*Full-Course Fitness Lean Legs and Gams Beginner Menu	
Day 1	*Day 3*	*Day 5*
Lunge (Chapter 10)	Lunge (Chapter 10)	Lunge (Chapter 10)
Outer Thigh Leg Lift (Chapter 9)	Resistance Band Squat (Chapter 10)	Legs Apart Thigh Flexion (Chapter 9)

Day 1	Day 3	Day 5
Inner Thigh Leg Lift (Chapter 9)	Legs Apart Thigh Flexion (Chapter 9)	Inner Thigh Scissor Cut (Chapter 9)
Legs Apart Thigh Flexion (Chapter 9)	Inner Thigh Scissor Cut (Chapter 9)	Standing Hip Abduction w/Band (Chapter 9)
Standing Heel Curl (Chapter 10)	Standing Hip Abduction w/Band (chapter 9)	Hamstrings Curl (Chapter 10)
Anytime Standing Saddlebag Toner (Chapter 9)	Hamstrings Curl (Chapter 10)	Standing Heel Curl (Chapter 10)
Standing Calf (Chapter 12)	Lifting Calf Seated (Chapter 12)	Sitting Calf Strengthener (Chapter 12)
Lifting Calf Seated (Chapter 12)	Raising One Leg Calf Lift (Chapter 12)	Standing Calf (Chapter 12)

Do an aerobic warm-up and end with a stretch. On days in between your tone-ups, do cardio. Eat sensibly.

Table 18-6	*Full-Course Fitness Lean Legs and Gams Advanced Menu	
Day 1	**Day 3**	**Day 5**
Resistance Band Squat (Chapter 10)	Lunge (Chapter 10)	Resistance Band Squat (Chapter 10)
Legs Apart Thigh Flexion (Chapter 9)	Great Legs Band Stretch (Chapter 10)	Legs Apart Thigh Flexion (Chapter 9)
Standing Hip Abduction w/Band (Chapter 9)	Standing Hip Abduction w/ Band (Chapter 9)	Great Legs Band Stretch (Chapter 10)
Inner Thigh Scissor Cut (Chapter 9)	Inner Thigh Scissor Cut (Chapter 9)	Outer Thigh Leg Lift (Chapter 9)
Standing Heel Curl (Chapter 10)	Outer Thigh Leg Lift (Chapter 9)	Standing Hip Abduction w/Band (Chapter 9)
Hams on a Bench (Chapter 10)	Hams on a Bench (Chapter 10)	Hamstrings Curl (Chapter 10)

(continued)

Table 18-6 *(continued)*

Day 1	Day 3	Day 5
Standing Calf w/Barbell (Chapter 12)	Raising One Leg Calf Lift (Chapter 12)	Standing Calf w/Barbell (Chapter 12)
Raising One Leg Calf Lift (Chapter 12)	Lifting Calf – Seated (Chapter 12)	Sitting Calf Strengthener (Chapter 12)

Do an aerobic warm-up and end with a stretch. On days in between your tone-ups, do cardio. Eat sensibly.

Shaping your abs and lower back

If you're serious about finally toning up your abs and strengthening your lower back, this menu is for you. It works all the core muscles, with the added benefit of improving your balance and stability. Focus on proper technique and breathing — always exhale on exertion. Beginners should check out Table 18-7, and advanced fitness enthusiasts should hit Table 18-8.

Table 18-7   *Full-Course Fitness Abs & Lower Back Beginner Menu

Day 1	Day 3	Day 5
Oblique Crunch (Chapter 13)	Lift and Cross (Chapter 13)	Side Waist Toner (Chapter 13)
Lift and Cross (Chapter 13)	Side Waist Toner (Chapter 13)	Oblique Crunch (Chapter 13)
Lower Abs Lift (Chapter 14)	Legs Up Lower Abs Lift (Chapter 14)	Seated Leg Lift (Chapter 14)
Seated Leg Lift (Chapter 14)	Seated Leg Lift (Chapter 14)	Lower Abs Lift (Chapter 14)
Crunch (Chapter 15)	Chair Lift (Chapter 15)	Wall Reach (Chapter 15)
Chair Lift (Chapter 15)	Wall Reach (Chapter 15)	Chair Lift (Chapter 15)
Pelvic Tilt (Chapter 16)	Dead Lift w/ Bent Knee (Chapter 16)	Pelvic Tilt (Chapter 16)
One Leg Lift (Chapter 16)	Pelvic Tilt (Chapter 16)	One Leg Lift (Chapter 16)

Do an aerobic warm-up and end with a stretch. On days in between your tone-ups, do cardio. Eat sensibly.

Table 18-8 *Full-Course Fitness Abs & Lower Back Advanced Menu

Day 1	Day 3	Day 5
Side Twist (Chapter 13)	Elbow to Knee (Chapter 13)	Crossed Leg Side Crunch (Chapter 13)
Crossed Leg Side Crunch (Chapter 13)	Crossed Leg Side Crunch (Chapter 13)	Side Twist (Chapter 13)
Belly Be My Best (Chapter 14)	Tummy Pull Leg Push (Chapter 14)	Bicycle (Chapter 14)
Legs Up Lower Abs Lift (Chapter 14)	Bicycle (Chapter 14)	Belly Be My Best (Chapter 14)
Toe Reach (Chapter 15)	Butterfly Lift (Chapter 15)	Belly Up (Chapter 15)
Butterfly Lift (Chapter 15)	Belly Up (Chapter 15)	Toe Reach (Chapter 15)
One Leg Lift (Chapter 16)	Superbeing (Chapter 16)	Lower Back Crunch (Chapter 16)
Lower Back Lift (Chapter 16)	Lower Back Crunch (Chapter 16)	Superbeing (Chapter 16)

*Do an aerobic warm-up and end with a stretch. On days in between your tone-ups, do cardio. Eat sensibly.

Firming your fanny

Hot buns can be yours with this intense menu. Twenty minutes or more, three times a week on alternate days can help zone in on this trouble spot. Beginners, start with Table 18-9; advanced folks, check out Table 18-10.

Table 18-9 *Full-Course Fitness Firming Your Fanny Beginner Menu

Day 1	Day 3	Day 5
Lunge (Chapter 10)	Lunge (Chapter 10)	Lunge (Chapter 10)
Squats (Chapter 11)	Squats (Chapter 11)	Squats (Chapter 11)
Anytime Standing Bun Burner (Chapter 11)	Resistance Band Squat (Chapter 10)	Resistance Band Squat (Chapter 10)

(continued)

Table 18-9 (continued)

Day 1	Day 3	Day 5
Resistance Band Squat (Chapter 10)	Anytime Standing Bun Burner (Chapter 11)	Anytime Standing Bun Burner (Chapter 11)
Floor Butt Lift (Chapter 11)	Great Legs Band Stretch (Chapter 10)	Floor Butt Lift (Chapter 11)
Bottoms Up Butt Lift (Chapter 11)	Floor Butt Lift (Chapter 11)	Bottoms Up Butt Lift (Chapter 11)
Great Legs Band Stretch (Chapter 10)	Bottoms Up Butt Lift (Chapter 11)	Kick Butt (Chapter 11)
Kick Butt (Chapter 11)	Kick Butt (Chapter 11)	Great Legs Band Stretch (Chapter 10)

Do an aerobic warm-up and end with a stretch. On days in between your tone-ups, do cardio. Eat sensibly.

Table 18-10   ***Full-Course Fitness Firming Your Fanny Advanced Menu***

Day 1	Day 3	Day 5
Lunge (Chapter 10)	Resistance Band Squat (Chapter 10)	Lunge (Chapter 10)
Squats (Chapter 11)	Bun Blast Off (Chapter 11)	Resistance Band Squat (Chapter 10)
Great Legs Band Stretch (Chapter 10)	Lunge (Chapter 10)	Squats (Chapter 11)
Kick Butt (Chapter 11)	Squats (Chapter 11)	Great Legs Band Stretch (Chapter 10)
Floor Butt Lift (Chapter 11)	Resistance Band Squat (Chapter 10)	Kick Butt (Chapter 11)
Bottoms Up Butt Lift (Chapter 11)	Anytime Standing Bun Burner (Chapter 11)	Floor Butt Lift (Chapter 11)
Squats (Chapter 11)	Kick Butt (Chapter 11)	Bottoms Up Butt Lift (Chapter 11)
Bun Blast Off (Chapter 11)	Bottoms Up Butt Lift (Chapter 11)	Bun Blast Off (Chapter 11)

Do an aerobic warm-up and end with a stretch. On days in between your tone-ups, do cardio. Eat sensibly.

Defining your arms

Both men and women look younger with toned-up, strong arms. This regular diet of biceps curls, triceps, and wrist moves can definitely define your arms. If you're a beginner, get started with the menu in Table 18-11. If you're advanced, you should check out Table 18-12.

Table 18-11	*Full-Course Fitness Arms Beginner Menu	
Day 1	*Day 3*	*Day 5*
Seated Same Time Biceps Curl (Chapter 8)	Lying Triceps Extension (Chapter 8)	Seated Same Time Biceps Curl (Chapter 8)
Angled Same Time Biceps Curl (Chapter 8)	Triceps Dip (Chapter 8)	Angled Same Time Biceps Curl (Chapter 8)
Seated Concentration Biceps Curl (Chapter 8)	One Sided Triceps Kickback (Chapter 8)	Seated Concentration Biceps Curl (Chapter 8)
Over the Head Triceps Extension (Chapter 8)	Over the Head Triceps Extension (Chapter 8)	Over the Head Triceps Extension (Chapter 8)
One Sided Triceps Kickback (Chapter 8)	Seated Same Time Biceps Curl (Chapter 8)	One Sided Triceps Kickback (Chapter 8)
Lying Triceps Extension (Chapter 8)	Seated Concentration Biceps Curl (Chapter 8)	Lying Triceps Extension (Chapter 8)
Triceps Dip (Chapter 8)	Angled Same Time Biceps Curl (Chapter 8)	Triceps Dip (Chapter 8)
Wrist & Reverse Wrist Curl (Chapter 8)	Wrist & Reverse Wrist Curl (Chapter 8)	Wrist & Reverse Wrist Curl (Chapter 8)

Do an aerobic warm-up and end with a stretch. On days in between your tone-ups, do cardio. Eat sensibly.

Table 18-12	*Full-Course Fitness Arms Advanced Menu	
Day 1	*Day 3*	*Day 5*
Seated Same Time Biceps Curl (Chapter 8)	Over the Head Triceps Extension (Chapter 8)	Wrist & Reverse Wrist Curl (Chapter 8)
Angled Same Time Biceps Curl (Chapter 8)	One Sided Triceps Kickback (Chapter 8)	Seated Same Time Biceps Curl (Chapter 8)

(continued)

Table 18-12 *(continued)*

Day 1	Day 3	Day 5
Seated Concentration Biceps Curl (Chapter 8)	Lying Triceps Extension (Chapter 8)	Seated Concentration Biceps Curl (Chapter 8)
Triceps Dip (Chapter 8)	Triceps Dip (Chapter 8)	Angled Same Time Biceps Curl (Chapter 8)
Lying Triceps Extension (Chapter 8)	Seated Concentration Biceps Curl (Chapter 8)	Lying Triceps Extension (Chapter 8)
Over the Head Triceps Extension (Chapter 8)	Angled Same Time Biceps Curl (Chapter 8)	One Sided Triceps Kickback (Chapter 8)
One Sided Triceps Kickback (Chapter 8)	Seated Same Time Biceps Curl (Chapter 8)	Over the Head Triceps Extension (Chapter 8)
Wrist & Reverse Wrist Curl (Chapter 8)	Wrist & Reverse Wrist Curl (Chapter 8)	Triceps Dip (Chapter 8)

Do an aerobic warm-up and end with a stretch. On days in between your tone-ups, do cardio. Eat sensibly.

Full-course circuit toning

This fun, fast-paced menu, in Table 18-13, of 20 minutes or more gets results. Each exercise is done one after another with no rest in between. You get the benefit of toning up your whole body while working your heart and lungs. (For more on circuit toning, see Chapter 17.)

Table 18-13 — Full-Course Circuit Toning All Levels Menu

Day 1	Day 3	Day 5
Shadow Box (1 min.)	Run in Place (1 min.)	Jump Rope (1 min.)
Flat Bench Press (Chapter 5)	Hamstrings Curl (Chapter 10)	Seated Same Time Biceps Curl (Chapter 8)
Bent Forward Row (Chapter 6)	Lunge (Chapter 10)	Over the Head Triceps Extension (Chapter 8)
Shadow Box (1 min.)	Run in Place (1 min.)	Jump Rope (1 min.)

Day 1	Day 3	Day 5
Deltoid Press (Chapter 7)	Great Legs Band Stretch (Chapter 10)	Oblique Crunch (Chapter 13)
Dumbbell Pullover (Chapter 5)	Inner & Outer Thigh Leg Lift (Chapter 9)	Tummy Pull Leg Push (Chapter 14)
Shadow Box (1 min.)	Run in Place (1 min.)	Butterfly Lift (Chapter 15)
Modified Push-up (Chapter 5)	Bun Blast Off (Chapter 11)	Pelvic Tilt (Chapter 16)

*Do an aerobic warm-up and end with a stretch. On days in between your tone-ups, do cardio. Eat sensibly.

Chapter 19

Discovering the Joy of Eating

*O*ur culture is constantly barraged with diet information — low-carbohydrate, high-protein, low-fat, low-calorie, eat this, don't eat that, and on, and on, and on. Every day you hear about some study or report that declares exactly the opposite of what you heard was true the day before. With all this conflicting information being spread through the airwaves, word of mouth, and cyberspace, it can drive you nutritionally nutty. This chapter intends to keep you sane with a simplified explanation of nutrition. In this chapter, I encourage you to bring back the joy of eating healthy and show you how to make smart and tasty food choices.

Making Food Work for You

Eating sensibly is very personal. That's why I deplore experts who claim that one diet or way of eating is right for everybody. What works for somebody else may not work for you. Have you ever had a friend who was all enthusiastic about a new way of eating, and when you try it, you gain weight or, worse yet, get sick? When you consider all the medical conditions such as diabetes, high cholesterol, or hypoglycemia, or any number of other health-related factors, it's no wonder formula fad food plans often fail. So, you have to discover a plan of what to eat and when to eat that's right for you.

Understanding the food groups

You need to maintain a sensible diet — as in, a pattern of eating for life, not a fad diet — in addition to working out to lose weight. With all the diet hype today, you may find it easy to forget that each day you need to include healthy servings of all the food groups in your diet — this makes for a sensible, varied diet.

As with any diet plan, you must discuss the changes you'd like to make with your physician to avoid any potential health problems.

You need to remember what food groups to include in your diet, how many servings, and what healthy choices can be made from those groups. To make this task I easier, I've listed all that information in the following sections.

I do recommend that you avoid certain foods in the following sections; however, I am not an advocate of depriving yourself of foods you love. Although you may want to indulge from time to time, moderation should be your mantra — keep your indulgences to a minimum.

Breaking bread (and other carbs)

The bread, cereal, rice, and pasta food group should be the base of your eating plan each day.

Having been born and raised in Detroit, and having worked as an auto show model, I can't help but draw this comparison: Your body is like the engine of a car, and carbohydrates are the fuel, or energy, that makes it run. Car enthusiasts carefully consider the quality of fuel pumped into their cars. What about the quality of your fuel intake — in other words, the food you eat? Complex carbs such as whole grains, bread, and pasta would be the "premium" fuel, whereas simple carbs like cakes, sodas, and pastries can be classified as "regular." Simple carbs may fill you up temporarily, but can cause you to run out of gas quickly (they unfortunately often stall out on your back bumper).

Basically, your diet should consist of 55 to 60 percent carbohydrates — which boils down to 6 to 11 servings — most of which should be the complex kind. Avoid simple carbohydrates, those that are higher in fat. A serving equates to one slice of bread or a half cup of cooked rice, cereal, or pasta. Just check out my recommendations that follow:

✔ **Healthy options:** Down some whole grains, hot cereal, dried peas, beans, plain noodle pastas, and whole grain pastas.

✔ **Unhealthy options:** Avoid daily doses of buttery crackers, muffins, doughnuts, and cream sauce on pasta.

Vegging out

Pros don't argue too much about the importance of this group because mom was right — you gotta eat your spinach, baby! You need three to five servings each day from this group. A serving is equal to 1 cup of raw leafy vegetables, ½ cup of cooked or raw veggies, or ¾ cup of vegetable juice. Vegetables are loaded with nutrients. Be adventurous and try all the different kinds you spot in the grocery store or farmers market. Try out my following suggestions:

✔ **Healthy options:** Choose green leafy vegetables, carrots, brussel sprouts, broccoli, squash, and cabbage. Raw or steamed vegetables are tasty on their own. You can even enhance the flavor with lemon juice or spices. Vegetable juices add a tasty zip over your favorite foods such as pasta or drink them on their own.

✔ **Unhealthy options:** You can't go wrong when choosing one vegetable over another — they're all healthy, but be sure to skip butter or cream sauce when you dress them up. See my ideas in the bullet above to find some flavorful alternatives to fatty sauces and creams.

Getting fixated on fruit

Getting in your fruits should be a priority on your list also. Although you don't need quite as many servings from this group each day — just two to four — this groups still constitutes an important part of your diet. Fruit is rich in vitamins, minerals and fiber. One serving is a medium-size apple, orange, banana, or pear; 1 cup of chopped, cooked or canned fruit; or 6 ounces of fruit juice. To make great choices with fruit, check out the following choices:

✔ **Healthy choices:** Try a medium-size apple, orange, or pear. Drink 6 ounces of orange, apple, or grapefruit juice. Nibble on a cup of your favorite berries.

✔ **Unhealthy choices:** Try to avoid fruits canned in heavy syrup, fruit drinks, and limit fruit juice to no more than 6-ounce servings.

If you have a sweet tooth like I often do, a fresh piece of fruit is very satisfying. When I was a little girl, my mother would freeze sliced peaches picked from a tree in our yard. They were yummier than any fattening pastry could ever be.

If counting your fruit and vegetable servings gets confusing, just remember the saying used by several health organizations: "Five a day." Five servings of fruit and vegetables are an easy way to make sure you meet the nutritional requirement.

Making the most of proteins

Meat, poultry, fish, dry beans, eggs, and nuts provide a nutritional staple in your diet — protein. Proteins are the building blocks of the cells and tissues in your body. You need them for a number of functions, including fluid balance, blood clotting, your immune system, and hormone production, among others. Experts banter back and forth as to how much protein you should consume. In general, it's safe to keep your protein intake at 10 to 15 percent of your daily calories, which constitutes two to three servings each day. A serving is equal to 2 to 3 ounces of cooked lean meat, poultry, or fish, ½ cup cooked beans, 1 egg, and ⅓ cup of nuts or seeds. To make the best protein choices, check out my following suggestions:

✔ **Healthy options:** Choose lean meats that are trimmed of fat and vary among beef, skinless poultry, and fish.

✔ **Unhealthy options:** Avoid deep fried meats and fatty cuts of meat, duck, organ meats, and sausage.

Skip foods that are deep fried or high in saturated fats. While restaurants may rave that their deep-fried meats, such as chicken, are low-carb, healthy choices, remember that low-carb doesn't necessarily mean low-fat or good for you. If the product is high in everything else, especially calories and saturated fat, pass over it for a healthier choice.

Milking the milk group for all its worth

Be sure to include this important food group each day also. It's rich in vitamin A, vitamin D, and calcium to maintain strong bones and teeth. Foods in this group provide proteins, carbohydrates, and if eaten in excess, too much dietary fat. You need two to three servings a day. One serving is equal to 1 cup of milk or yogurt, 1½ ounces natural cheese, 2 ounces processed cheese, or 1½ cups of ice cream. Following are some great choices:

✔ **Healthy options:** Select foods such as low-fat and non-fat cheese, skim or low-fat milk, low-fat yogurt, and low-fat cottage cheese. Choose fat-free items from this group. That way you miss the saturated fat while consuming important nutrients.

✔ **Unhealthy options:** Avoid whole milk, cream, and a serving of ice cream the size of a pint.

Making good choices with fats, oils and sweets

This group of fats, oils, and sweets should be a miniscule part of your daily diet. The USDA doesn't even give a recommended serving amount for this group because the group includes all the foods that are high in fats and simple sugars (cake, cookies, doughnuts, pies, and candy). The message is loud and clear: Use sparingly. My following suggestions should steer you in the right direction:

✔ **Healthy options:** Use light virgin olive oil for cooking or to top pasta instead of creamy sauces. You can also munch on some unsalted nuts — just a handful, as well as a small portion of olives.

✔ **Unhealthy options:** Avoid foods, such as brownies, cupcakes, soda, candy bars, coffee cream flavors, frosting, butter, and so on.

To reach your health and fitness goals at a fast pace, cut back on calories. But rather than cutting out sweets altogether, try a more gradual method. For example, fat intake should not be higher than 30 percent of your daily calories. If you usually go way overboard on fat, cut back gradually by a more livable 5 percent. That way you are more likely to succeed.

Keeping a food journal

During the day it's easy to be unaware of what you're eating, but a food journal monitors not only everything that goes into your mouth, but also when you eat and why. The food journal can monitor your eating patterns and aid in altering your behavior for faster results. The key is to jot down everything you eat, including all the snacks — no cheating! Boy, do they add up! Journaling everything about what and how you eat keeps you focused on your immediate goals and serves as an excellent kick-start to carry you long into the future. Why not continue to use the skills you are developing now to shape a long-term healthier lifestyle?

If you include the following in your food journal, you can discover your eating patterns, whether they're healthy, and how you can change them for the better:

- ✔ **Food:** In this section, jot down all the foods you eat for breakfast, lunch, dinner. Remember not to skip those snacks. You have to know what you're eating so you can figure out if you need to start limiting certain foods or incorporating other foods that you need.

- ✔ **Time:** Record what time it is each time you eat. This information, coupled with how you feel (see the next bullet) can show you when you're actually hungry and needing food during the day. You can then structure meals and snacks around this info.

- ✔ **Emotion:** Make a note of what you are feeling when you eat. For example, are you tired? Frustrated? Calm? Are you actually hungry? This valuable information can show you if you're falling into negative eating patterns so you can opt for positive ones.

- ✔ **What/Where:** Write down what you are doing while you are eating and where you are. For example, you may be watching TV or reading a newspaper while munching on potato chips in a waiting room. Doing so can show you places where you may be vulnerable to unnecessary snacking.

- ✔ **Calories:** Record the amount of calories consumed for each food item. Add the total calories for each meal, for all the snacks, and a grand total for the whole day. You might want to be sitting down when you do so. Noting which foods put you over the nutritional edge shows what you need to start limiting or cutting out of your daily diet. If you are not using pre-packaged food that has the calorie information printed on the label, pick up a handy pocket calorie counter from any bookstore. It can help you become more aware of how many calories you are consuming.

- ✔ **Nutrition check-up:** Tally up your servings for each food group (see earlier in this chapter for the different food groups and their recommended servings). A quick glance at this area in your food journal can not only tell you what you're missing each day, but it can also serve as a handy way to make healthier decisions each day. For instance, if you're hungry and need a snack, see how many servings of each food group you have left. Knowing you have some extra milk and fruit servings to get in may steer you toward an apple and some low-fat yogurt and away from the latte and brownie.

Getting Yourself to Lighten Up

If excess weight is dragging you down and is no longer a funny matter, it's time to lighten up. You really can cut calories without being deprived of food, especially foods you love. Just by cutting out a smidgen here or a smidgen there, you can trim down at a healthy, safe, fast pace. Gradual weight loss is the safest way to go, and most studies show that steady weight loss is more likely to stay off. In other words, subtle changes are more likely to get lasting results. So cut a few calories here and there to lighten up and you can have the last laugh!

Following are some simple tips to help you lighten up for good:

- ✔ Substitute nonfat milk for whole milk.

- ✔ Try turkey chili with beans, rather than beef chili with no beans.

- ✔ Use a nonstick pan spray when greasing a pan.

- ✔ Marinate raw veggies in low-cal Italian dressing for a delicious snack. Cover and keep in the refrigerator. You can nibble all day.

- ✔ Make a great low-cal dip by using plain yogurt mixed with spices.

- ✔ Spread toast with fruit jam instead of butter for breakfast.

- ✔ Serve your salad on a large plate and your main meal on a smaller plate.

- ✔ Prepare your fish poached with a little juice.

- ✔ Have a small slice of pizza when you get the urge, rather than the regular jumbo size.

- ✔ Substitute a whole candy bar when you're craving chocolate with one small truffle, and discover the pleasure of savoring it slowly.

- ✔ Chew sugarless gum instead of regular.

- ✔ Measure a level tablespoon of salad dressing for your greens instead of the usual three to four. You probably won't even miss it.

- ✔ Get one scoop of ice cream instead of two.

Chapter 20

Adding a Cardio Workout

• •

In This Chapter

▶ Discovering the benefits of cardio workouts

▶ Getting the scoop on aerobic exercise

▶ Selecting a cardio workout

▶ Finding your target heart rate

• •

*B*eing in shape is much more than pumping up a bicep muscle and striking a pose in the mirror. It also requires more than sucking in your gut when someone walks by who you want to impress. To be physically fit, you need to work on your strength, flexibility, *and* cardiovascular (cardio) endurance. Adding a cardio workout to your program can really accelerate your results and has tremendous health benefits. (See Chapter 2 to review fitness testing, and Chapters 17 and 18 for pre-packaged fitness menus that can meet your needs.)

In this chapter, I show you how to lose the fat by adding a cardio workout and I provide several aerobic choices to suit your individual preferences. I explain how you can determine what your target heart rate is and offer tips on how to take your pulse. All of this gets you moving toward a successful cardio workout.

Using Cardio for Maximum Benefits

When you do tone-up exercises, or any kind of weight training for that matter, you are actually strengthening and shaping up your underlying muscles. But after working so hard to achieve your muscle definition, why hide it under layers of fat? Doing an aerobic activity such as running, walking, or dancing helps burn calories to cut through the fat. (See Chapter 1 for more on the importance of replacing fat with firm muscle.)

In addition to looking good, you can expect a cardiovascular workout to help you feel better and improve your overall general health. I've often thought that if nonexercisers gave cardio workouts an honest try, they would feel so good they wouldn't want to stop. Aerobic exercise strengthens your heart so that it can pump blood at a steady pace and allows your lungs to breathe better — that means you can get through your day like a dynamo with energy to spare. A cardio workout can also lead to lower blood pressure and cholesterol and helps prevent heart disease and a number of other illnesses. If you want to look and feel better fast, this chapter gets to the heart of it.

Leaving Your Legwarmers in the Closet

The term *aerobics* often conjures a vision of women jumping up and down to music by The Pointer Sisters. Wearing pink tights, legwarmers, and a matching sweat band may have been left behind in the '80s, but an aerobic workout is just as important today. We now know that there are huge benefits to performing safe, large, rhythmic moves and that they don't have to destroy your joints in the process.

Aerobic means "with air," whereas *anaerobic* means "without air."

For health purposes, both aerobic and anaerobic workouts are necessary for your system. When you do the exercises in this book, your body is working anaerobically. That's because you are taking a rest between exercises and are using stored energy. The circuit tone-ups are somewhat aerobic because you move from one movement to the next without a rest (for more on circuit toning, see Chapter 17). Before you pooh-pooh the idea of an aerobic activity as some girlie thing from the past, consider this: Any movement that goes longer than a minute and a half requires oxygen for the muscles to work in an aerobic way. That means you can choose among any number of activities, including the classic aerobics workout, to fulfill your aerobic requirement. Running, jogging, or riding a bicycle are a few examples of other cardio activities. Aerobic activity can strengthen your heart and lungs and improve your cardiovascular fitness — something both men and women need.

Experts recommend 30 minutes of cardiovascular activities daily. If it is not realistic for you to schedule that kind of time, studies show that it can be beneficial to do ten-minute sessions throughout the day. Walk during a coffee or lunch break or pedal a bike in front of the TV. You can also choose to do a longer aerobic activity on days between your ten minute tone-ups.

Many beginners are overzealous and overdo cardio workouts. Remember that the heart is a muscle. If you are just starting out or haven't exercised in a while, do an aerobic activity for no more than 10 to 20 minutes at a time. You can gradually increase to 30 minutes or more.

Choosing a Cardiovascular Workout

You can choose from a ton of cardiovascular workouts. Finding something that you *enjoy* doing makes your workouts more enjoyable and more success-ful. You are then more likely to stick to it. Many people experience a natural high from the increased circulation. Hang on to that feeling to help you face the day with all its ups and downs. I've provided some great cardio choices along with tips to help you move like a pro, but feel free to come up with your own aerobic selections.

It's important to breathe when exercising. This is particularly true when doing a cardiovascular workout, which is based on the flow of oxygen. Never hold your breath.

For safety reasons, always do a cardio workout within your target heart rate range. I explain how to determine what that range is and how to stay there in the section "Finding your target heart rate" later in this chapter.

Always warm up before doing a cardio workout. Start out and end at a low intensity level.

Power walking

I love power walking. First of all, it's free. It can be done anywhere and it puts very little pressure on the joints. Whether you use a treadmill, sneak out your front door, or cruise the shopping mall, strutting your stuff is a safe and effec-tive cardio workout. It can do amazing things toward taking one's disposition from bad to good. I also find that it instills creativity. I probably wrote half this book in my mind during my daily walking ritual.

When walking, stand tall. Hold the abs in tight. Keep the shoulders back, but down. Pump your arms back and forth at a 90-degree angle. Push off through your heels. Keep your face looking forward, not down (review Chapter 1 for posture pointers).

When walking at night, it is safest to wear light-colored or reflective clothes.

Riding a stationary bike

The stationary bike can provide a very effective cardio workout. A number of excellent ones are on the market (see Chapter 3 for more on home equip-ment). Using a stationary bike that has moveable handlebars can provide the added benefit of an upper-body workout. Take the time to imagine being in the country, the mountains, or even the beach. A ride on your bike can help you escape while delivering aerobic results.

Your seat should be adjusted so that when your legs are in the down position there is a slight bend in the knees. Use the handlebars for light support, but do not lean into them with all your weight. Keep your shoulders relaxed.

As you pedal, keep your knees forward, and not out to the side, to avoid injury. Keeping your knees in a side, frog-like position can irritate the joints and eventually cause pain.

Shadow boxing

Shadow boxing is a fun way to work off steam and accomplish a cardio workout at the same time. Jab, punch, right hook, left hook — it doesn't matter if you don't know Oscar De La Hoya from Oscar De La Renta or Oscar Mayer Weiner, just as long as your body is moving in large, rhythmic motions. Imagine you are beating down all your troubles. Shadow boxing can help you to manage your stress while you get all the benefits of a super cardio workout.

Dancing

If dancing puts you in the groove, let it take you to your personal best aerobic heights. Turn on the radio, CD, or MP3 player and just keep moving. Choose music that is upbeat and energizing. Chapter 3 has more on how to select music to move and motivate you.

Use large movements to move your arms and legs. This can get the circulation going throughout your entire body and raise your heart rate.

Jumping rope

Men and women of all ages enjoy jumping rope. It is an activity that can make you feel young at heart. Pull out that jump rope and feel like a kid again as you burn calories and work your heart. If you find it too challenging to jump non-stop, take a ten-second break every ten seconds until your endurance improves. Be patient.

Feel free to do this aerobic activity minus the rope if you are a beginner, haven't exercised in a while, or are just a klutz. It's easier, but still very effective. You can do all kinds of fancy skips and steps because it's impossible to trip on an imaginary rope! (If you trip anyway, you can pretend it's part of your routine — I won't tell.)

Workout step or stairs

Going up and down stairs provides an excellent cardio workout. You can use a workout step that is available at any sporting goods store (see Chapter 3 for more on exercise equipment) or the stairs at your home, office, park, or mall. The up and down motion is a great way to get the circulation going and work the heart. For best results, pump your arms during your workout.

The bonus "behind" this type of workout is a great set of buns.

Don't bend or lean forward from your waist during the up and down movement so as not to take your back out of neutral alignment (review Chapter 1 for posture tips).

Be Not Still My Beating Heart

Many experts say that when you do vigorous exercise, you should stay within your target heart rate zone (also called your training heart rate zone). This is excellent advice! You've heard it before, but what in the world does it mean? Your target heart rate zone is the range where your heart and lungs get the best workout — and the safest. This is important, because if you're working below your training zone, you are not going to get any results, whereas working above your training zone can be dangerous.

Finding your target heart rate

Your training heart rate range should fall somewhere between 60 percent and 85 percent of your maximum heart rate. Your maximum heart rate is the highest heart rate you individually can achieve during vigorous exercise. Don't panic! I'm going to tell you how to figure this out.

First, subtract your age from 220. This is your maximum heart rate. Multiply your maximum heart rate by .6 (60 percent) to find the lower end of your target heart rate zone. Then multiply your maximum heart rate by .85 to find the higher end of the zone. You now have your target heart rate zone. This is where you should be during exercise. For example, if you are 36 years old, your target heart rate zone is 110 to 156 beats per minute. Let me show you how that is determined:

1. 220 minus 36 years old is equal to 184. This is the maximum heart rate.

2. 184 times .6 equals 110, the lower end of the training zone.

3. 184 times .85 is 156, the upper end of the training zone.

4. The target heart rate zone for a 36-year-old during exercise is between 110 to 156 beats per minute.

If you are a beginner or haven't exercised in a while, it is safest to exercise near the lower range of your target heart rate. Always start and end your cardio workout in the lower end of the range to serve as an aerobic warm-up and cool-down.

You can check yourself during exercise by counting the beats of your pulse for ten seconds. Multiply the number of beats by 6 and see if that number falls within your training or heart rate zone. If it's too low, you've got to work harder. If it's too high — slow down. I explain how to check your pulse later in the section "Taking your pulse" later in this chapter.

Another safe intensity-level indicator is being able to carry on a normal conversation while doing your cardio workout.

Taking your pulse

Taking your pulse properly can prove to be beneficial during a cardio workout. You can monitor the intensity of the activity and adjust your workout level accordingly to meet your individual needs. You can also keep track of your progress. The following is the least amount of information you need to know about your pulse.

Finding your pulse

If you are usually searching in vein for your pulse, don't get frustrated — let me explain. It is fine to use either your wrist or neck — whichever is easiest for you. Take the pads of your index and middle fingers and press down on the wrist of your opposite hand. With your hand facing upward, feel the base of your thumb. Take your fingers and slide them down to about an inch below the thumb base. Press gently until you feel your pulse. To take your pulse on your neck, raise your chin up and feel for a pulse next to your Adam's apple.

Do not press the pads of your finger so hard that you restrict blood flow to your hand or head.

After you feel your pulse, watch the second hand of a clock as you count your heartbeats for ten seconds. Your counting should start with zero, not one. Take the number of heartbeats and multiply by six to arrive at your heartbeats per minute.

Knowing when to take your pulse

Knowing when to take your pulse can immediately improve your cardio workout. Take advantage of this on-the-spot tip. During an aerobic activity, it is best take your pulse about 5 minutes into your workout session. If you discover that you haven't reached your target heart rate, increase the intensity of your activity and re-check your pulse in another 5 minutes. Once you reach your target heart rate, stay there until it's time to cool down.

Stop the exercise or decrease the level of difficulty if you are breathless or unable to carry on a normal conversation.

Check your pulse after cooling down to find out what your resting heart rate is. As you become more fit, it takes less time to return to your resting heart rate.

Peddling pedometers!

Let's hear it for pedometers! These are nifty little devices that can count your individual footsteps by monitoring the up and down movement of your body. They are small and are worn on the hip. Every time you move, they go click, click to count your steps. The average person takes 10,000 steps a week, which equates to 3,500 calories — one pound of fat in terms of calories. Watching the numbers on the pedometer add up quickly can inspire you to keep moving. You can pick up a good one at any sporting goods store for as low as $25. Some well-known brands include New Lifestyles and Yamax.

Chapter 21

Traveling Fit and Well

Traveling, whether for business or pleasure, is often met with its share of mishaps and stress. This chapter is filled with all kinds of great tips to help you stay healthy on the road — even if you don't have a lot of time. I explain how to prepare for a fit trip, including what to pack, and offer the secrets to a relaxing yet energizing journey. Once you reach your destination, I show you how you can incorporate exercising into your traveling schedule and share the healthy do's and don'ts of dining out on the road. You may forget a toothbrush, socks, or your underwear, but after applying the tips from this chapter, you won't forget to travel fit and well.

Preparing for a Healthy Trip

Half the fun or drudgery (depending on your perspective) of going on a trip is preparing for it. Taking the time to plan ahead can make your life on the road easier. This section is loaded with helpful information on packing healthy snacks and first-aid information as well as a handy fit-trip checklist. Because scheduling a workout at home can be challenging enough, it's even more critical to make your traveling fitness plans as convenient as possible.

Using the fit-trip checklist

Use this nifty fit-trip checklist to help you leave town on the road to wellness:

- ✔ **Call the hotel before you arrive to see about a gym:** If you are staying in a hotel, try to find one that has a gym. Not all hotel gyms are created equal. Some have state-of-the-art, full-facility spas, whereas others consist of nothing more than one beat-up bike. You can also ask the hotel operator for the name of a nearby gym. Many gyms offer privileges for hotel guests.

- ✔ **Pack workout garb:** Always throw something in your suitcase that you can move in. Sweat pants, t-shirt, shorts, and a sweatshirt are easy to pack. Don't forget the gym shoes. I travel so much that when I return from a trip I automatically replace my worn workout wear with a fresh set that I keep in my suitcase. If a last-minute trip comes up, there is no way I leave without my fitness garb. (Unless I take a different suitcase — okay, it happened once. I resorted to working out in my room.)

- ✔ **Consider the weather:** Don't get caught out of town with nothing more than a sleeveless muscle tank or jog-bra top. These items may shine on a hot sunny day, but they don't fair well should the temperature drop. Since out-of-town fitness often takes you outside, opt for clothes that you can layer (see Chapter 24, where I list my top ten favorite workout wear manu-facturers). I like to log on to www.weather.com before I travel. Punch in the city you are going to for the most up-to-date weather information.

- ✔ **Bring workout tapes/DVDs:** Many hotels offer in-room VHS or DVD play-ers. Take advantage of this service whenever you can. There are a number of tapes that work great in a limited amount of space. Yoga and Pilates tapes are especially nice when there is not much room. My favorite collec-tion of fitness tapes comes from Collage Videos. Call (800) 433-6769 to get a copy of its catalog or log on to www.collagevideo.com. If you are stay-ing with friends, you can bring a tape/DVD along, and all of you can join in. Leave it there as a thoughtful gift.

- ✔ **Take a reward:** Always travel with something that is personally reward-ing to you. I never leave town without a candle and bubble bath. These are simple little pleasures that I look forward to after my out-of-town workout. You might enjoy a favorite mystery novel or old-fashioned sta-tionery to write to a loved one. The calming effect is just as important for health as any workout can be. It can also keep you motivated and able to manage stress better (see Chapter 2 for more on rewarding yourself).

- ✔ **Pack tubing and bands:** Exercise tubing and bands are perfect for trav-eling. They offer resistance, take little space, and fit neatly in a suitcase (see Chapter 3 for more on exercise equipment).

Exercising out of town

When out of town, it's easy to use traveling as an excuse not to exercise. This is a grave mistake, because adding fitness into your schedule can enhance the experience of your business or pleasure trip. You may not be able to work out at the same gung-ho pace you can at home, but even a little movement can boost your energy level. This can help your meetings become more successful and your sightseeing more enjoyable.

You can get a cardio workout simply by walking or jogging out the hotel door. Ten minutes are better than nothing. It helps to talk to the concierge to make sure the neighborhood is safe. He or she will often have a handy map ready to give to you with a highlighted route, including some pretty neat points of interest. Enjoy the surroundings of a new environment as you briskly move. If the outside grounds make you feel uncomfortable, use the hotel stairs or check to see if the hotel has a treadmill or exercise bike.

While you are inside the room, take at least ten minutes to tone up each day. Be sure to take the anytime-anywhere menu I provide for you in Chapter 17. These exercises can be done anywhere in a minimum amount of time. If you are feeling more ambitious, pull out your exercise tubing and resistance bands — they travel well (see more on exercise equipment in Chapter 3). You can also use hotel items as makeshift weights if you like — hairdryers, towels, or a business attaché that you may have brought with you. Try doing your favorite fitness menu from Chapters 17 or 18 — most of the exercises work perfectly in a hotel room. If you keep this up, you can take your goal beyond 30 days into a lifetime of fitness. Now *that* travels well!

Eating out healthy

Half the fun of traveling is enjoying the culinary delights of the town you are visiting. There is no need to totally deny yourself these tempting pleasures as you try to eat out healthy. With a little common sense, you can tantalize your taste buds by making sensible choices.

When dining out at a restaurant take the time to carefully read the menu. Select foods that are steamed, roasted, or broiled. Avoid foods that are fried, sautéed, or have been creamed because they are loaded with fat and calories. Don't be afraid to request to have your food prepared in a way that is not on the menu. For example — if I see sautéed spinach on the menu, I ask to have it prepared steamed, without the butter. I can always add pepper or other spices if I choose. Dress it up without the extra calories. Most chefs are happy to make these changes.

Fast food is often unavoidable on the road. Fortunately, many fast food restaurants have introduced the option of healthier fare. Ask to see a nutritional information sheet if you aren't sure what is the healthier choice. Avoid combo meals, sauces, and anything fried. Choose fruit salads, turkey, or lean ham sandwiches without the mayo. Even a regular hamburger is better than the triple decker that many places offer. (Review Chapter 19 for more tips.)

Packing healthy snacks

Traveling can lead you to bad nutritional temptation. It goes with the territory. You may have vending machines stocked full of super-size candy bars, coupled with midnight hunger pangs. Usually, no one can see when you indulge. Many rooms have a stocked bar at the foot of the bed that, I swear, chants, "yummm — eat me!" Short of performing an exorcism, you can banish the evil by being prepared. Pack convenient, healthy, portable snacks. I say *pack* because sometimes a busy schedule doesn't allow for nutritional snack shopping away from home. I take along packages of dried fruit and nuts that are already distributed in a healthy portion size. It's too easy to consume too many calories without even realizing it. Size does matter (see Chapter 19, where I explain serving sizes). Energy bars are nice, too. However, read the labels — some have more sugar than a candy bar.

When I'm out of town on business, I am often invited to evening functions. At a recent convention where I was promoting my fitness videos, I was invited to one cocktail party after another, followed by a late company dinner. In situations like that, rather than starve myself beforehand to save my appetite for dinner, I consume a snack just before I walk out the hotel room door. Many times, I pack a small jar of reduced-fat peanut butter in my suitcase. I put a tablespoon (not a jar!) on an apple or a banana. It gives me an aura of energy and helps me resist the surplus calories often available at social functions. When dinner is finally in front of me, I can eat sensibly rather than scoffing up everything in sight. I have a wonderful time without widening my waist.

Packing first aid

Recent research shows that 60 percent of people say they get sick when traveling. That's not counting medical mishaps such as cuts, bruises, and scrapes. The experienced traveler knows the importance of packing a first-aid kit. Here's a list of items to include in your kit that can help you stay well when away.

  ✔ **Take your medication:** This is so basic but probably one of the most frequently forgotten items. Always remember to pack your medication and take extra, just in case your trip is prolonged for some reason. It also helps to keep the phone numbers of your doctor and pharmacist in your day planner. That way you can contact them if you run out.

✔ **Pepto-Bismol:** If an upset stomach hits you, there is nothing like the pink pill. Remember to brush your tongue of the cotton candy color before attending any out-of-town welcome reception.

✔ **Sun block:** Wear sun block when out of town to protect your skin. Even if you are just driving, and are not fully outside, the sun's damaging rays can still hit you through the windows of your car. Make sure your sun block has a minimum SPF of 15 and covers a wide spectrum of both UVA and UVB rays.

✔ **Pain medication:** Slip some aspirin or Tylenol in your bag. Traveling often lends itself to its share of aches and pains. Besides, if you see the price of two pills in a pack at the hotel gift shop, you are *sure* to get a headache — and maybe pass out from sticker shock.

✔ **Insect repellent:** This is a must-have for any outdoor, camping, or wildlife trip. I wonder if they also make a repellent for hotel lounge lizards and barflys?

✔ **Bandages:** Take along varying sizes, perfect for cuts, scrapes, and broken nails.

✔ **Antibacterial treatment:** I always travel with an antibacterial treatment for emergency cuts. Neosporin is my favorite. It helps to prevent scarring.

✔ **Antibiotics:** Talk to your doctor about an antibiotic if you are going to a country that has bacterial agents in the water.

✔ **Decongestant and nose spray:** If your nose becomes congested, this can make your trip much more bearable.

✔ **Superglue:** I always pack superglue, because nothing repairs a broken nail like this neat invention. Okay — it's not a real emergency item, but I always take it anyway.

Keeping Fit in Flight

Flying fit and well is within your reach with the following tips. The sky's the limit if you follow these guidelines:

✔ **Move around:** Do not stay frozen in one position while on an airplane. If you don't have to climb over too many people, get up and walk around every hour or so. At the very least, do exercises from your seat (shoulder rolls, stand up and stretch, rotate ankles).

Leg movements help prevent vein thrombosis, a serious blood-clotting condition. The clot can sometimes travel to your lungs. Some people with this problem need to wear compression stockings — consult with your physician.

✔ **Breathe:** Flying nowadays is met with many fears — terrorism, turbulence, and a terrible 2-year-old sitting next to you. Realizing that flying is probably the safest way to travel may not always calm you down. Taking slow, deep breaths is a great way to enhance your journey. I remember taking off from LAX one time when, 30 seconds into the air, the left wing caught on fire. Fear filled the cabin. I began taking slow, deep breaths to calm me down. During a situation that was out of my control, I continued to breathe deeply until we had a safe emergency landing in Ontario, California.

✔ **Chewing gum:** If you experience ear pain while flying due to cabin pressure, chew gum. Swallowing can also help if you forget to bring gum. Have young children drink from a bottle to keep their ears open.

✔ **90-degree knees:** Try to sit tall while in flight to maintain good posture. It helps to keep your knees bent at a 90-degree angle because that automatically puts your hips into a healthy 90-degree angle for back safety. If you are petite like me, you can rest your feet on your carry-on luggage under the seat in front of you.

✔ **Drink water:** The recycled air in a plane can be extremely drying. Take every opportunity you can to stay hydrated. Avoid caffeine when flying.

✔ **Use vegetable oil:** If you experience nasal dryness when you fly, dab a little vegetable oil under your nostrils. This secret ingredient can make your flight more comfortable, especially in the dead of winter. However, vegetable oil under the nostrils does not constitute a serving of vegetables (see Chapter 19 for vegetable serving information).

✔ **Plan for plane meals:** When on a plane, the meal options are not always the best. In fact, nowadays you are lucky if you even get a meal. However, if food is served, some airlines let you order special meals ahead of time (kosher, vegetarian, low-fat). The best option is to prepare your own food. Pack a tasty turkey sandwich, apple, and a handful of nuts or raisins.

Driving Fit

Road trips by their very nature tend to make many throw caution to the wind. I recently took a fun-filled trip across the country in my little red sports car. I playfully refer to the trip as "my wild and free tour." Thankfully, I know how to drive fit. Below I share a few of my secrets:

✔ **Snack healthy:** Sitting in a car for hours does not give you an excuse to gobble up junk snacks, unless you intend to pack on the pounds. (Review the section "Packing healthy snacks" earlier in this chapter for yummy alternatives.)

✔ **Take a stretching break:** Stop every hour for a stretching break. It's important to actually get out of the car for fresh air and to energize. If you are the driver, this is particularly true for safety reasons. Run, jump, bend, and stretch. Do something that gets you moving.

✔ **Carry water:** Drink plenty of water while you drive. This can help you avoid becoming dehydrated.

✔ **Don't slouch:** Try to maintain good posture on a car trip. I realize this is not always easy, but you can avoid back pain later if you skip slouching. Place a small pillow behind your back to help keep your spine straight. Use cruise control to relieve pressure.

✔ **Exercise in the car:** Squirm, wiggle, squeeze your buns, and move your body every time you can. This can prevent stiff shoulders and cramped legs. Obviously, for safety reasons you should wait till your car is at a complete stop and traffic permits. If you are driving, always keep both hands on the wheel. For a fun selection of exercises you can do from a seated position in your car, home, or office, order a copy of my audio-tape "Drive to Fitness" (Starglow) by logging on to my Web site `www.starglow.com`. The program can tone your body and improve posture. It includes a segment that helps to manage stress and instills a positive mental attitude. Exercising in your car can energize you so that you are more alert.

Taking Action Vacations

When planning a vacation, why not choose one that is action-packed? I'm not talking about a week of James Bond movies. There are numerous trips that can keep you moving (hiking, river rafting, biking tours). Even cruise lines these days offer more than dessert buffets. When I lectured for Royal Caribbean Cruise line, passengers left with healthy lifestyle tips to take home. There was a gym, and trainers were on board, and there were tasty, healthy cuisine choices with each meal. Perhaps you can try a spa vacation for yourself or with a loved one. Imagine a weekend of pampering and fun-filled healthy activities! These and other options are available for you to travel fit and well.

Part VI
The Part of Tens

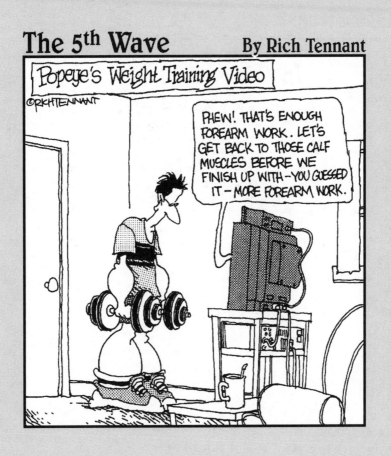

Popeye's Weight Training Video

©RICHTENNANT

PHEW! THAT'S ENOUGH FOREARM WORK. LET'S GET BACK TO THOSE CALF MUSCLES BEFORE WE FINISH UP WITH—YOU GUESSED IT—MORE FOREARM WORK.

In this part . . .

1 get to share with you some of my top-ten lists to make you feel like a "10." Because motivation is such an important element to a successful program, I've charted out ten common motivational pitfalls and how to avoid them. You can also find ten ways to fit a toning session into your busy schedule — no more excuses! And check out my personal picks for where to get great workout wear for men and women.

Chapter 22

Ten Common Motivational Pitfalls

Motivation — it's that spark that drives one to achieve dreams and goals, an attitude that pushes through obstacles with a vengeance, and an unscathed determination to succeed. What is the secret of those who have captured this elusive spirit? How can you personally use motivation to take your fitness goals to new heights for life? In this chapter, I've gathered lots of tips that can help you reach your target date with the confidence of a peacock. So here are ten common motivational pitfalls that can crush you if you let them. Don't let them. You have the power within yourself to take these tips and make them work for your ultimate well being.

An amazing side effect can happen if you take these tips to heart. Embracing motivation can go way beyond a 30-day tone-up target date (see Chapter 2 for more on creating your 30-day target date). We all need to constantly motivate ourselves. Everything from finishing a college degree, raising children, meeting your sales quota at work — even getting out of bed in the morning sometimes — all take motivation. Heck, I needed it to complete this chapter. Accepting our human frailty helps us overcome all the motivational pitfalls that come our way. Embrace this information as the ammunition it takes to tone up for your target date and to survive triumphantly all the challenges of life (see Chapter 2 for some more suggestions on how to get and stay motivated).

Low Self-Esteem

Having low self-esteem can be detrimental to achieving your fitness goals. Let's put it this way: If you think that you cannot win, you have already lost — and I'm not talking about your weight. A self-defeating attitude does nothing but set you up for failure. If you suffer from low self-esteem, you might ask yourself what caused it. With a 30-day target date, you don't have time to be glum and pessimistic about your life (see Chapter 2 for more on creating your 30-day target date). Pick yourself up by your boot straps and get into some serious self-improvement. It helps to realize that each of us is unique. If you don't see yourself *already* as an individual worthy of self respect, toning up won't make a difference. Take time to value your worth. Self-esteem is not predicated by the size of your wallet or the number on a scale. It is measured by the size of your heart, and how much you love and respect yourself and others.

Body Image Problems

Have you looked in the mirror recently and gone — yuck!? Everybody does that on occasion, but if you do that regularly, there is a good chance you suffer from a body image problem. You're not alone, research shows that 58 percent of women and 43 percent of men are dissatisfied with their appearance, and 66 percent of women and 52 percent of men are constantly dissatisfied with their weight. What is most interesting is the dissatisfaction that both men and women have with their body parts. Seventy-one percent of women and 63 percent of men dislike their mid torso. 61 percent of women and 29 percent of men dislike their lower torso, and 34 percent of women and 38 percent of men dislike their upper torso. An astounding 57 percent of women and 45 percent of men wish they had better muscle tone.

What's compelling is that both men and women are suffering from body image problems. The difference seems to be that women are more likely to talk about it. Men tend to keep it inside. This is not really that surprising when you think of all the perfect images and extreme makeovers being presented to us everyday. It's not just average Joes who suffer this debilitating problem, but even models, celebrities, and athletes who appear to have it all. I know a gorgeous model who has posed several times in gentlemen's magazines. By all accounts, she is pretty close to perfect. Yet every time she looks in the mirror the only thing she sees is her cellulite. Deep down she is troubled by the finished photos because she knows her cellulite has been digitally touched up in the pictures.

It's healthy to care about your looks. However, it becomes dangerous when the way you perceive yourself becomes distorted. If you aren't careful, it can even lead to eating disorders. Looks should never be a complete measurement of your self worth.

Review "Loving your naked self — yes, really!" in Chapter 2. It has pointers that can help you appreciate the body you have been given. Flip further through the pages of Chapter 2 to have a better understanding of how genetics contribute to realistic goals. Find out your body type and how muscle fibers affect your results. Go forward with confidence that you can be your personal best.

Lack of Time

Lack of time is probably the biggest excuse that people give for not exercising. Guess this is a sign of our hurried times. Technology and a world of so-called modern conveniences are supposed to make life simpler for us, but so often it seems just the reverse. Everybody is rushing. It used to be that when you got to your office, you checked your messages from an assistant or coworker. Now we deal with cell phones, voice mail, e-mail, faxes, videoconferences, and on and on, and that's all before your first cup of coffee in the morning and just after putting the baby down in your home office. Well, take a deep breath and hear this: Exercise can *give you more energy* to complete all those tasks and thus *save* you time.

For more information on how to schedule a ten minute, 30-day workout, see Chapter 2. Chapter 23 is also jam-packed with ways to fit fitness into your schedule.

Significant Other Leaves You

Loosing a significant other when a relationship falls apart or through death can be an extremely devastating experience. Life may seem to no longer have meaning. The thought of exercising, or anything else for that matter, may be the last thing on your mind. If your emotions are out of control, and you can't function, be sure to seek professional help.

When it comes to matters of the heart that have left you feeling hurt or angry, try practicing what I call "controlled crying." Give yourself permission to cry or scream till you get it out of your system. It doesn't change the situation, but helps you handle it better.

As you go through your healing process, it really does help to exercise. Exercise helps relieve stress. Be kind to yourself during this difficult time.

Long Hours at Work

The traditional eight-hour workday seems to be a thing of the past. It's not unusual for people to leave for work at the crack of dawn, spend long hours sitting at a desk, and sit as they drive home late in the day or early evening.

How easy it is to let your life go by without the healthy benefits of exercise. Don't let long hours at work be a motivational pitfall for you. Here are some great suggestions:

✔ **Do the anytime-anywhere menu:** Take advantage of the handy Time Crunch menu in Chapter 17. These exercises are perfect to take to work.

✔ **Pack a fast-fitness menu for lunch:** Make your favorite **fast-fitness** menu from Chapter 17 a part of your next lunch meeting. Change off each day for variety. You can store a few weights or resistance bands at your desk or use objects at work.

✔ **Work out before driving home:** Drive home relaxed after a workout and avoid the rush hour.

✔ **Exercise in your car:** Simple shoulder rolls or bun squeezes are helpful at stop signs and red lights (see Chapter 21 for more on car-trip tips).

✔ **Move when you can:** Take the stairs rather than the elevator. Don't e-mail that coworker down the hall — walk to her cubicle. Park your car in the farthest spot.

Mental Fatigue Versus Physical Fatigue

One of my clients was having a horrible time sticking with her workout routine when I wasn't with her. I questioned her, and she said that every time she went to work out she was "just too fatigued." Upon further investigation, I found out that she was studying for an intense course in college, and her mind was being taxed to the limit. Well, of course: Hours and hours of studying left her mentally fatigued. Her mind was exhausted. That is different from physical fatigue when your body gets tired, but it's very easy for mental fatigue to leave you feeling drained and not very excited about doing a workout.

When you recognize mental fatigue, use it as a motivating signal to take tone-up time. Exercise uses oxygen to get the circulation going in your body. This wakes up the brain and ultimately wakes you up. That's why I always do a power walk before writing — to eliminate any mental fatigue. It wakes up my brain and my body.

Distraction Excuses

"Just a minute, I'll be right back, I've got to get the phone." "Excuse me, it's the door." "Once the kids get back to school, I'll start my routine." "My mother-in-law is moving in. It'll just have to wait." "I can't possibly begin an exercise regime with so many emotional problems." These are just a few of the many distraction excuses that can prevent you from toning up. It's easy to procrastinate from doing your exercises. I had a client who came to me after unsuccessfully maintaining any fitness schedule. Before our meeting I had asked her to keep track of her daily physical activities. Upon review, it became apparent that she was spending an enormous amount of time house cleaning. Now, I knew she wasn't a professional housekeeper, and she had just mentioned how bored she was with her small two-bedroom apartment. Something wasn't adding up. I questioned her about this, and a light bulb went off. She realized that her obsession with over-cleaning her apartment was detrimental to not only missing out on the benefits of exercise, but living life to her fullest potential. She had lots of other goals as well, and her distraction excuses prevented her from achieving many things. Within a month, she was feeling great from working out and well on her way to finishing a painting that she had started long before.

Try to identify what your distraction excuses are. From there you can focus on changing your pattern. Review your activity log for concrete evidence of where and how you can change (see Chapter 1 for suggestions on how to create and use an activity log).

Non-supportive Influences

This is a really big motivational pitfall, and I mean big. Non-supportive influences can psychologically destroy any positive move forward unless you cut them off at the pass. See if you recognize any of these negative influences in your own life, and if so, try to address them:

- **Spirit crushers:** Spirit crushers are those people who try to zap your positive energy. Many times on the surface they seem to be friends or people who care. Everybody has felt the sting of a backhanded compliment. "Gee, Mary, you look great since you started working out. You spend so much time at the gym, I bet your husband is looking elsewhere." Comments like this may be said with a smile, but they can hurt. Spirit crushers usually have other issues going on. Perhaps they are jealous of you or feel inadequate with themselves. That doesn't matter so much, though, because the "why" is out of your control. What matters is how you react to situations involving an unsupportive person.

Start becoming aware of spirit crushers in your life and recognize the way you feel around these people. It helps to surround yourself with a sincere support system. To help you build a positive team, see Chapter 23.

- **Your own inner demons:** If you are not supportive of yourself and your fitness goal, it can be difficult to maintain a healthy regime. It may even be more of a challenge to put together a positive support system. If you don't believe in yourself, why should anyone else? Spend a little time addressing the issues that may be preventing you from believing in yourself. Is it low self esteem? Body image? Review both of these topics earlier in the chapter. Once you jump on your own bandwagon, others will follow.

✔ **Substance abuse:** Abusing drugs and alcohol can be a major non-supportive influence. If you have been in denial of inappropriate use of substances, now is a great time to make a positive change. Fitness can work in synch with your rehabilitation. Seek help from a professional, a rehab clinic, or Alcoholics Anonymous.

Cost Factors

If you were to base the success of any workout on having to use costly treadmills from TV infomercials, joining expensive gyms, or going to health spa weekends in the Caribbean, you might be justified in thinking that cost was a motivational pitfall. These luxuries may be beneficial to those who can partake, but they are poor excuses to not get in shape. Let me scream out loud and clear: Fitness is *free!* I doubt that the cavemen, pioneers, and western frontiersmen struggled with what the cost of a health club membership was going to be, but they were probably in great shape. You can succeed at achieving your fitness goals for the inexpensive cost of this book.

Minimal equipment is needed to achieve your ten minute tone-ups goals. Check out Chapter 3 where I provide inexpensive alternatives.

Take advantage of several ways to incorporate free fitness into your life. You can run in the park, take the stairs at work, play baseball, soccer, or badminton, to name a few examples.

Lack of Will Power

Lack of will power is a leading motivational pitfall. There are a ton of reasons why people lack the will power to maintain a health and fitness regime. To help you make it to your 30-day target date (see Chapter 2 for more on creating your 30-day target date), I've provided some suggestions that can keep you zipping along.

✔ **Review your tone-up contract:** If you signed the Ten Minute Tone-Ups commitment contract in Chapter 2, now is a good time to review it. If you didn't sign it, you may want to consider doing so now to boost your will power.

✔ **Use variety:** Incorporating variety into your workout schedule can eliminate boredom and escalate your enthusiasm. Check out the **fast-fitness** and full-course fitness menus in Chapters 17 and 18. Mix them up for variety and tone-up success.

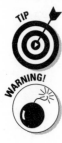

✔ **Dress confidently:** Sometimes dressing in a style that makes you feel good about yourself can help to light a fuse. Check out all the workout manufacturers in Chapter 24. Discover what style works best for you in appearance and function.

✔ **Get plenty of rest:** Sleep is an underrated component of a successful fitness program. The amount necessary varies from individual. If you experience constant sleep deprivation, be sure to contact a sleep disorder specialist.

✔ **Discover motivation techniques:** There are tons of ways to improve your will power. Discover which technique works best for you. Review Chapter 2 where I give you tips to help you get and stay motivated.

✔ **Hire a trainer:** Sometimes having a professional trainer can encourage will power. Try to look for someone who is certified by a professional organization such as ACE, AFAA, ACSM, or NSCA. It helps if he or she has a degree in exercise science, anatomy and physiology, or kinesiology. Just because someone has a buff body does not make him or her knowledgeable enough to meet your needs.

✔ **Find a workout buddy:** Working out with a buddy can sometimes help to keep you on track. See how to find a good one and what type works best for you in Chapter 23.

Chapter 23

Ten Ways to Fit Tone-Ups into Your Schedule

*W*hen I was a little girl my father used to tell me that health was the most important thing in life. I didn't understand what he meant. My mind bubbled with thoughts of peace, love, and harmony. How could health be more important than any of that? Well, anyone who has suffered a serious illness or experienced a loved one's pain and limitations through sickness or death understands this concept. Dad has passed on since then, but I can still hear his voice. He taught me in his life, as well as his death, that health truly is our most valuable asset.

Whether your goal is to tone up in 30 days for an event or establish a lifetime commitment to health, scheduling daily ten minute tone-ups requires time-management skills. It's so easy to get caught up in our busy lives. How many times have you put together a "to-do" list and never got to the "doing" part? In this chapter, I help you explore ways to fit ten minute tone-ups into your schedule. I show you how to prioritize and I explain the benefits of sometimes leaving things unfinished. You can discover which technique works best for you — perhaps you need a workout buddy, for example. You can also try logging activities in a journal or toning up as a family or group activity. I also suggest how to schedule fitness as a part of an entertaining activity. There are also useful tips to help you remember to do your ten minute tone-ups. You can even discover your personal optimum fitness time and create a support system that builds you up with positive energy all through the process.

Prioritizing

It is often said that if you want something done, ask a busy person. Successful business men and women, dynamic homemakers, and people who pull off both roles all have two things in common: They are busy and they prioritize. You can incorporate your ten minute tone-ups into your life with a little of their wisdom. Follow these suggestions:

✔ **Make a "to-do" list:** Most people have heard about to-do lists, but how many actually put one together? Don't let your mind get cluttered with things that need to be done — get them on paper. A list frees your mind for other creative avenues, such as deciding what to wear to that upcoming reunion to show off your new shape.

A to-do list works best if you make a new one every day. Insert "do ten minute tone-ups" each day in your planner pad or PDA to serve as a visible call to action.

✔ **Prioritize items:** Place your most important goals at the top of the list and try to accomplish these first. Schedule your ten minute tone-ups as a priority. Avoid doing unnecessary or routine items (reading your horoscope, playing video games) first because that can keep you from accomplishing projects that are a top priority, such as exercise. It's easy for these activities to distract you from achieving your goals. For more on distracting excuses, see Chapter 22.

✔ **Not doing it all:** If you are very busy, you may not be able to do the whole list. Accept this condition as an opportunity to make a new list for the next day. I discuss leaving certain things unfinished in the next section. Always try to accomplish your top priorities, including the ten minute tone-ups.

Leaving Things Unfinished

Sometimes it's just more effective to leave things unfinished (have you ever heard of Franz Schubert's *Unfinished Symphony?*). I am by no means suggesting that you not complete your ten minute tone-ups. I am suggesting that not finishing other things that aren't as important may afford you more time to complete the high-priority items more effectively. For example, writing this book has brought with it some tight deadlines. I made a conscientious decision to make that a priority. Therefore, my desk is not as neat as it could be — cleaning has been left unfinished. Are there mundane things in your day-to-day life you can keep unfinished so that you can schedule your ten minute tone-ups (see "Prioritizing" earlier in this chapter)?

Finding a Workout Buddy

Can a workout buddy help you stick to your ten minute tone-ups schedule and get great results? It depends on the type of buddy.

- ✔ **Avoid a bad buddy:** A bad buddy constantly makes excuses to skip a workout, such as shopping or just being too tired. He or she may spend the whole session talking, which exercises your jaw but not much else. And it's not unusual to be coerced into going out afterwards for something fattening to eat. Boot the bad buddy bye-bye.

- ✔ **Getting a good buddy:** Getting a good buddy is a great idea. The camaraderie can help both of you stick to the schedule. If you slip, he or she encourages you, and vice versa. Together, you eat healthy, stay active and committed, and offer each other helpful tips.

Entertaining Fitness

Who says fitness has to be boring? To stay enthusiastic, you can make it more entertaining. Do your ten minute tone-ups while watching a favorite DVD or video, for example. Many people enjoy running on a treadmill or peddling a stationary bike while reading *The Wall Street Journal* or a romance novel. Use your MP3 player or a headset and CD player to listen to your favorite music. Or perhaps an audio book. In any case, entertainment can distract you from becoming overly conscious of what your body is doing.

Toning Up as a Family or Group Activity

Because you are probably not isolated on top of a mountain, you might find that family and friends can make it harder for you to fit exercise into your schedule. It's healthy to balance your life with fun family outings and social interaction with friends. Spending quality time with your loved ones is priceless. These people *should* be a priority. Show them that you care about them as well as yourself by scheduling fitness together. This is a healthy choice that can benefit all involved. Here are some suggestions:

- ✔ **Ten minute tone-ups together:** Squeezing in ten minute tone-ups may be less difficult if you get a whole group involved. In fact, it can be a blast. (Try using the fast-fitness menus in Chapter 17 or, for a longer tone up, the full-course fitness menus in Chapter 18. Take turns leading the group with a favorite menu. You can also each pick a different exercise to create a custom-made circuit tone-up, where you quickly move from one exercise to the next — always a group hit! Review Chapter 17 for circuit tone-ups tips.

✔ **Fun activities:** Getting together with family and friends doesn't have to mean you all become couch potatoes. There certainly is nothing wrong with delving into deep, profound thoughts with your loved ones while you sit on the sofa. However, how much richer the conversation can be after a planned physical activity! Your mind is stimulated after exercise, and your body feels good. Think about going out dancing with friends or taking the family on a hike. Try racquetball or a favorite sport.

Even just going out for a walk after dinner is helpful. Last Thanksgiving, I was at the home of one of my sisters and her husband. Afterwards, a group of us went out for a brisk walk. There are almost 30 of us in my immediate family and that's not counting aunts and uncles. Although not everybody went walking, you can imagine the sight of this huge family pack. We had a wonderful time and did not suffer the typical feelings of being over-stuffed.

Logging Your Activities

One of the best ways to schedule fitness into your life is to log your activities. I discuss this further in Chapter 1, along with other ways to boost your activity level. Be as specific as you can with your log. Jot down everything you do, from walking at the mall to doing your ten minute tone-up sessions. Don't forget to write down the time spent on all activities. Use this logged information to help you increase your activity level and chart your progress.

One way to increase your activity level is to take the stairs when you can instead of the elevator. And rather than going up one step at a time, go up two steps at a time. I always do this at my home, which has three levels of stair-stepping fitness. The plus is: It can give your butt an extra boost!

Making a Support System

There is nothing like the dynamic energy and enthusiasm that can come from being surrounded by a positive support system. A team that believes in you and offers unstoppable encouragement can take your health and fitness goals to new heights. You can start to build your ten minute tone-ups team by removing non-supportive influences in your life, such as spirit crushers, your own inner demons, or substance abuse (I show you how to identify these motivational pitfalls in Chapter 22).

I personally make every attempt to surround myself with positive people and energy. This is not an "everything is rosy" tendency, because that's not real. What I mean is you should try to surround yourself with genuine people who love you enough to pump you up with words of encouragement to help you be your personnel best — now *that's* real. Let your support system inspire you to adhere to your ten minute tone-ups schedule.

Using Reminders

Tying a string around your finger is not the only way to remember to schedule your ten minute tone-ups. The secret is to discover what works best for you. Oh — before I forget, here's a list of other suggestions to fit in fitness:

✔ **Trip on your equipment:** I have a friend who keeps her tone-up equipment smack dab in the middle of her living room. Exercise bands, weights, and a floor mat are there when she first wakes up. They don't get put away until she completes her tone-ups. At night, she brings them out again.

✔ **Tell a friend:** My friend Jennifer swears that just telling somebody that you tone up every morning or evening helps keep you accountable. Different from a support system, having someone at work remind you that you said you're going to work out each evening after work can nearly shame you into doing it! You hate to come in the next day and say, "No, I didn't tone up!"

✔ **Leave yourself a note:** Notes to yourself make wonderful reminders. Post-its indeed are an ingenious invention. Use them or scratch paper to remind yourself to schedule tone-up time! Place them on your wall, desk, refrigerator, or forehead if you have to — they work.

✔ **Use technology:** Have fun with today's technological advances. Send yourself an e-mail as a reminder — or a cell phone text message that you don't delete till you tone-up. Have a friend send you an instant message at a prearranged time. Get up from that computer and move! I know a guy who has a microwave he can program to talk. Pop in a pizza, and the microwave says "tone up."

✔ **Keep tone-up stuff handy:** Be prepared by always keeping a gym bag in your car or workout stuff in your desk. Just don't let them sit there — use them.

Discovering Your Personal Optimum Fitness Time

One of the best parts of ten minute tone-ups is that it can be done wherever and whenever you want. You may wonder when is the best time to schedule them to get optimum results. Some experts push morning workouts as if they were the only option. That's fine if you are a morning person and your schedule allows for it. It can even give a sluggish person more energy in the early hours of the day. However, if you are so slow in the morning that your techniques and form are off, it might be better to tone up later in the day. Your workout sessions will be more effective if you do them when you are at your best. Consider what time of the day fits best into your life schedule, as well as when your body responds most efficiently. That's your optimum fitness time.

Say No to Others

Sometimes taking time for yourself can cause others in your life to get upset because it takes attention away from them. Try these suggestions.

- **Just say no:** This can sometimes be the hardest word to say in the dictionary. Nobody wants to appear rude and uncaring. However, there are situations when other people can have you doing things that are simply a waste of your time. Become comfortable with a straight *no* or a simple apology that explains you are busy.

- **Make a compromise:** Sometimes a straight no doesn't feel right, especially if it's a child, best friend, or significant other. This is where making a compromise can be helpful. For example, say your son is begging to go see the latest hot movie, but you want to tone up. To save time, have him fold the laundry and do a few other chores you need done. This frees you to tone up, gets the chores done, and you can both enjoy the movie.

Scheduling "flex time"

Setting an appointment time with yourself in your daily calendar to exercise can help with exercise adherence. However, more often than not life throws us a curve, and things change. Scheduling what I call "flex time" offers you a backup. You can always fall back on this extra time slot. Being flexible ensures success. Try scheduling your back-up flex time for after dinner. Because it's later in the day, you can always have one last chance for exercise or a ten minute tone-up session.

Chapter 24

Ten Favorite Workout-Wear Manufacturers

• •

In This Chapter

▶ Discussing workout wear

▶ Choosing workout wear

▶ Buying workout wear

• •

People constantly ask me, "Where did you get that workout wear? I love it!" As a model involved in fashion, I've developed a keen eye for style. However, when it comes to workout wear, I'm a stickler for products that are functional and of the best quality (see Chapter 3 for more on workout wear). Whether you are a man or woman, looking your best and finding products that function well when you work out goes beyond what the scale says. Whatever your size, age, or pocket book, you have several great choices. I've scouted fitness conventions and industry trade shows to find the latest, newest, coolest, and absolute best workout-wear manufacturers. Here are my favorites in random order.

Everlast

When one thinks of the company Everlast, professional boxers usually come to mind. After all, it was Jack Dempsey who was the first champion to wear the Everlast label on his trunks and gloves. Since then, hundreds of fighters, including Joe Louis, Muhammad Ali, and Sugar Ray Leonard have worn the Everlast brand. It's no surprise that Everlast has lived up to its name and has serviced the boxing industry for more than 90 years. What you may not know is that you and I can dress like a champ, too, without even fighting. Everlast has a complete line of men's and women's workout apparel as well as accessories that can make you look and feel like a total knockout.

The young men's sportswear includes velour suits, fleece sets, and varsity jackets. Men of all ages can also choose between t-shirt tops, warm-up suits, and workout pants. The elastic-waist workout trunks, made out of 100 percent cotton jersey, are ideal for working out or casual wear. They also come in large sizes that are loose but neat looking on men, as opposed to just plain sloppy. (See more on workout wear in Chapter 3.)

The women's line is really neat, too. Everything from t-shirts to workout shorts to warm-up suits, all with the famous Everlast band. They are very comfortable and durable.

The entire workout-apparel collection has a comfy, tough-chic look about it. That just means you don't have to be a boxer or have a perfect body to wear it. You will also feel confident when toning up. Trends come and go, but if you're looking for quality, it's got to be Everlast.

Everlast products are available at several retail locations, or shop at the Web site www.everlast.com.

Hot Skins

The name says it all. If you want to feel like you rule during your ten minute tone-ups, Hot Skins workout wear sizzles. Designed by Trish Sereda for men and women, you can feel her passion for making the human form look its best. She is beloved by fitness pros for her inner warmth and her creative spirit. Trish was honored with the prestigious "Designer of the Year" title at the Academy of Bodybuilding, Sports, and Fitness Awards. She may dress the best bodies in the world, but Hot Skins fits most everyone who tones up. Hot Skins guarantees its body contouring fit to be the best you've ever worn. The company uses power hold fabrics to flatter and support the body and also use wider, draw cord, elastic waists to keep you secure during any workout.

Ten years ago, Trish invented the "body shaped" cut to follow the natural curves of the body. For example, the shorts and tights are slightly bigger in the thighs and calves, so you don't have to keep pulling on the fabric when working out. No more sagging areas.

Guys love Hot Skins. It was one of the first companies to get men to wear Lycra (that stretchy fabric). That's because the stitching is so good; men are not afraid that the material might separate.

Personally I, like many women, love the endless mix-and-match possibilities that Hot Skins gives to my workout wardrobe.

It's true that lots of fitness pros flaunt their stuff on TV, magazines, and in competitions donning Hot Skins. Well, now the secret's out — you can strut, too! For more information visit www.hotskins.com or call 800-468-0065.

Nike

Dressing athletes, fitness professionals, and the average Joe on the street, Nike is known for classic, quality workout wear. I've always been a big fan of Nike shoes. In fact, at the yearly IDEA World Fitness Convention, I always stop at the Nike booth to find out what's hot. The Nike shoes are very popular because of their superb stability, grip, flexibility, and impact protection. Enjoy the many styles that Nike has to offer. There is something for every sport or activity, and they have even designed a shoe that imitates the bare-foot runners of Kenya. However, whatever the style, always try on the shoes and look for a pair that fits your particular foot type. Review Chapter 3 where I discuss searching for the right shoes.

Active women enjoy wearing Nike. It offers everything from undergarments to workout tops, shorts, pants, skirts and dresses in fabrics that are functional and comfortable. I often sport its cute but practical jogging suits. This way I can layer for a day of activity. It's not unusual for me to power walk in my suit, run errands and then zip off the jacket and pants to uncover my workout wear.

Guys like Nike apparel because they provide "real" clothes for "real" men. Who can deny the comfort of a basketball tank or a t-shirt made out of Nike Sphere fabric (polyester knit) that doesn't cling and keeps sweat away from the skin. Choose to look neat in their pants or shorts made from a loose but stretchy Dri-FIT Fabric that allows you to stay cool and dry. Of course there is also tons of stuff in fleece to make movement easy. Feel free to lounge in these very livable garments. After a good tone-up session, you deserve it! For more information about Nike products, visit any of its retail outlets or check out www.nike.com.

Blue Fish

Blue Fish is a manufacturer of upscale active wear. It has produced cutting-edge women's workout wear since 1998. I can't say enough about Blue Fish's high-tech fabrics, captivating colors, and functional designs. They are very stylish and chic. Inspired by the Latin culture and hotter than hot Brazilian fashions, Blue Fish is not for the mild-mannered woman. This apparel says "I want to get noticed." Whether you are running on the beach, flexing at the gym, or burning calories on the dance floor, Bluefish easily moves from your ten minute tone-ups to the streets and beyond.

Each Bluefish garment is designed with superior craftsmanship. Every piece is colorfast and exceptionally comfortable. It's known to keep its shape while absorbing excess moisture. For more on Bluefish activewear, visit any of its retail outlets or www.bluefishactivewear.com.

New Balance

New Balance got its early start in 1934 selling arch supports to policemen and others who had to stand for long hours. Arch supports and prescription footwear were the mainstay until 1961, when the company introduced the revolutionary Trackster. The Trackster was the world's first performance shoe, featuring a triple sole and available in several widths. It became a hit with college running coaches and fitness directors. Till this day, that same quest for quality is in all of its products.

I like that New Balance focuses on function over fashion in all of its shoes. It makes them stylish in an earthy sort of way. They are proud of their "Endorsed by no one" stance, and they should be.

If you have a problem with shoe fit, remember: New Balance comes in multiple widths. For more information, visit www.newbalance.com.

Oxygen

Oxygen is a leading manufacturer of women's active wear. They specialize in high-tech fitness and yoga apparel. Their products are made out of Supplex, by DuPont, which makes them very livable, breathable, windproof, and wrinkle-proof. The styles are sexy, but not too sexy, meaning women of different sizes can wear them and feel confident. Hey, if you're doing your ten minute tone-ups, you should be confident!

If you are pregnant and looking for some maternity workout wear, Oxygen makes some fabulous pants, shorts, and tops. For more on Oxygen, visit www.oxygenfitnesswear.com.

Freddy

If you have a funky, fun personality, Freddy fitness wear may be for you. For men and women, it has a hip urban feel that shouts attitude. Freddy has everything from shoes to athletic jackets and from tanks to rhinestone camisoles. The craftsmanship is beautiful, and the designs come from Italy.

Because Freddy is an Italian manufacturer, it uses the European sizing system. Don't worry, you can call the toll-free number, and a customer rep can help you determine your correct size. For more information, call toll-free 866-330-1338 or point your browser to www.freddy.com.

Budget workout wear

Being on a budget does not mean that you can't look and feel good about yourself. There are plenty of places that you can find high-quality, hot-looking workout wear to match your personality and pocket book. Here are my three favorite budget workout wear retailers:

Target: I love this place, with its aisles of workout wear that are reasonably priced and high quality. For more information, check out www.target.com.

Wal-Mart: Famous for its smiley face, rolled-back prices, and friendly service, Wal-Mart is a welcome source of fitness fashion. Lots of comfy workout stuff. I spotted several cute Danskin items, all reasonably priced. For more info, try www.walmart.com.

Kmart: Buys are to be found at Kmart. Guys can snap up sharp, sporty tops and bottoms by Athletech for a steal. For more info, visit www.kmart.com.

Reebok

When it comes to a top ten workout *anything*, you cannot leave out Reebok. Since 1890, Reebok has been servicing athletes with quality products. In fact, it was in 1924 when the original family-owned business made the running shoes that athletes wore in the Summer Olympic Games, so beautifully portrayed in the movie *Chariots of Fire*. When I wear Reebok, I like the lateral support it gives my ankles, as well as the flexibility it offers in the forefoot. Reebok makes stable shoes with good shock-absorption qualities. Of course, its apparel holds its own as well.

For more information, visit www.reebok.com.

Thorlo

I can't say enough good stuff about Thorlo socks. They are designed to protect your feet from the constant abuse you get from the effects of impact and thereby help prevent blisters that are common in workouts. They are so comfy and cushiony, I can't help but rave about them. Guess you'll just have to try them out for yourself. For consumer inquires, call 888-THORLOS or visit www.thorlo.com.

Thorlo socks have three levels of protection. It is recommended that you wear them when you purchase new shoes, because you might need a pair of shoes one-half size larger.

Under Armour

If you are serious about quality workout wear, Under Armour is one of the best. It's a leading manufacturer of performance apparel for both men and women. Its garments are made to withstand any kind of weather condition. Under Armour uses an exclusive microfiber fabric that wicks sweat from your skin so that your body can adjust to the temperature no matter what's going on with the elements.

Many men clamor for the heatgear full or sleeveless tee. Both provide more coverage and support than traditional muscle tank tops or tees. They are comfortable and enhance a man's shoulders no matter what his size. Like a second skin, they are designed to keep you cool and dry. Many guys also like the fleece pants since they have built in power stretch panels to improve mobility. Another big plus are the side seem split pockets. You can carry lots of stuff (keys, change, license etc) and still get your workout done.

Women can feel confident during any sports activity when wearing an Under Armour sports bra. I particularly like the designs that have stitching that criss-crosses the chest for additional support. You can pair any of its tops with a huge selection of bottoms such as capris, shorts or long pants all made out of fabric built to last and last. You can find Under Armour at many retail outlets or visit its We site at www.underarmour.com.

Workout-wear Web sites

Here are a couple of really neat Web sites that offer workout wear from a bevy of manufacturers. Have fun shopping in the comfort of your own home or office — it could save you even more time to do your ten minute tone-ups.

www.usbodyware.com: Shop for fitness wear by several manufacturers from around the world without ever leaving your easy chair (except to do your ten minute tone-ups). Even if you don't buy, it's always fun to window shop.

www.sandiegofit.com: This site specializes in women's workout apparel. It's a favorite because it caters to every body type, including plus sizes, maternity wear, and more. Lots of great manufacturers to choose from.

Index

• **F** •

• *G* •

USINESS, CAREERS & PERSONAL FINANCE

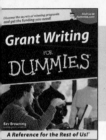

0-7645-5307-0

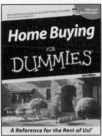

0-7645-5331-3 *†

Also available:
- ✔Accounting For Dummies †
  0-7645-5314-3
- ✔Business Plans Kit For Dummies †
  0-7645-5365-8
- ✔Cover Letters For Dummies
  0-7645-5224-4
- ✔Frugal Living For Dummies
  0-7645-5403-4
- ✔Leadership For Dummies
  0-7645-5176-0
- ✔Managing For Dummies
  0-7645-1771-6

- ✔Marketing For Dummies
  0-7645-5600-2
- ✔Personal Finance For Dummies *
  0-7645-2590-5
- ✔Project Management For Dummies
  0-7645-5283-X
- ✔Resumes For Dummies †
  0-7645-5471-9
- ✔Selling For Dummies
  0-7645-5363-1
- ✔Small Business Kit For Dummies *†
  0-7645-5093-4

OME & BUSINESS COMPUTER BASICS

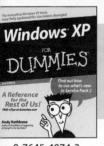

0-7645-4074-2

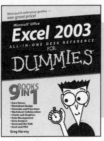

0-7645-3758-X

Also available:
- ✔ACT! 6 For Dummies
  0-7645-2645-6
- ✔iLife '04 All-in-One Desk Reference
  For Dummies
  0-7645-7347-0
- ✔iPAQ For Dummies
  0-7645-6769-1
- ✔Mac OS X Panther Timesaving
  Techniques For Dummies
  0-7645-5812-9
- ✔Macs For Dummies
  0-7645-5656-8

- ✔Microsoft Money 2004 For Dummies
  0-7645-4195-1
- ✔Office 2003 All-in-One Desk Reference
  For Dummies
  0-7645-3883-7
- ✔Outlook 2003 For Dummies
  0-7645-3759-8
- ✔PCs For Dummies
  0-7645-4074-2
- ✔TiVo For Dummies
  0-7645-6923-6
- ✔Upgrading and Fixing PCs For Dummies
  0-7645-1665-5
- ✔Windows XP Timesaving Techniques
  For Dummies
  0-7645-3748-2

OD, HOME, GARDEN, HOBBIES, MUSIC & PETS

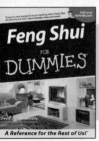

0-7645-5295-3

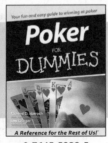

0-7645-5232-5

Also available:
- ✔Bass Guitar For Dummies
  0-7645-2487-9
- ✔Diabetes Cookbook For Dummies
  0-7645-5230-9
- ✔Gardening For Dummies *
  0-7645-5130-2
- ✔Guitar For Dummies
  0-7645-5106-X
- ✔Holiday Decorating For Dummies
  0-7645-2570-0
- ✔Home Improvement All-in-One
  For Dummies
  0-7645-5680-0

- ✔Knitting For Dummies
  0-7645-5395-X
- ✔Piano For Dummies
  0-7645-5105-1
- ✔Puppies For Dummies
  0-7645-5255-4
- ✔Scrapbooking For Dummies
  0-7645-7208-3
- ✔Senior Dogs For Dummies
  0-7645-5818-8
- ✔Singing For Dummies
  0-7645-2475-5
- ✔30-Minute Meals For Dummies
  0-7645-2589-1

TERNET & DIGITAL MEDIA

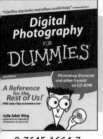

0-7645-1664-7

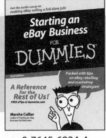

0-7645-6924-4

Also available:
- ✔2005 Online Shopping Directory
  For Dummies
  0-7645-7495-7
- ✔CD & DVD Recording For Dummies
  0-7645-5956-7
- ✔eBay For Dummies
  0-7645-5654-1
- ✔Fighting Spam For Dummies
  0-7645-5965-6
- ✔Genealogy Online For Dummies
  0-7645-5964-8
- ✔Google For Dummies
  0-7645-4420-9

- ✔Home Recording For Musicians
  For Dummies
  0-7645-1634-5
- ✔The Internet For Dummies
  0-7645-4173-0
- ✔iPod & iTunes For Dummies
  0-7645-7772-7
- ✔Preventing Identity Theft For Dummies
  0-7645-7336-5
- ✔Pro Tools All-in-One Desk Reference
  For Dummies
  0-7645-5714-9
- ✔Roxio Easy Media Creator For Dummies
  0-7645-7131-1

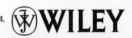

SPORTS, FITNESS, PARENTING, RELIGION & SPIRITUALITY

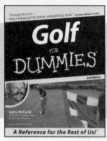

0-7645-5146-9

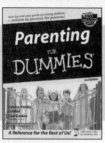

0-7645-5418-2

Also available:
- Adoption For Dummies
  0-7645-5488-3
- Basketball For Dummies
  0-7645-5248-1
- The Bible For Dummies
  0-7645-5296-1
- Buddhism For Dummies
  0-7645-5359-3
- Catholicism For Dummies
  0-7645-5391-7
- Hockey For Dummies
  0-7645-5228-7

- Judaism For Dummies
  0-7645-5299-6
- Martial Arts For Dummies
  0-7645-5358-5
- Pilates For Dummies
  0-7645-5397-6
- Religion For Dummies
  0-7645-5264-3
- Teaching Kids to Read For Dummies
  0-7645-4043-2
- Weight Training For Dummies
  0-7645-5168-X
- Yoga For Dummies
  0-7645-5117-5

TRAVEL

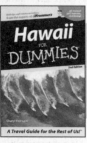

0-7645-5438-7

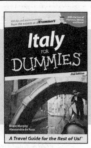

0-7645-5453-0

Also available:
- Alaska For Dummies
  0-7645-1761-9
- Arizona For Dummies
  0-7645-6938-4
- Cancún and the Yucatán For Dummies
  0-7645-2437-2
- Cruise Vacations For Dummies
  0-7645-6941-4
- Europe For Dummies
  0-7645-5456-5
- Ireland For Dummies
  0-7645-5455-7

- Las Vegas For Dummies
  0-7645-5448-4
- London For Dummies
  0-7645-4277-X
- New York City For Dummies
  0-7645-6945-7
- Paris For Dummies
  0-7645-5494-8
- RV Vacations For Dummies
  0-7645-5443-3
- Walt Disney World & Orlando For Dummies
  0-7645-6943-0

GRAPHICS, DESIGN & WEB DEVELOPMENT

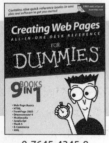

0-7645-4345-8

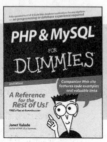

0-7645-5589-8

Also available:
- Adobe Acrobat 6 PDF For Dummies
  0-7645-3760-1
- Building a Web Site For Dummies
  0-7645-7144-3
- Dreamweaver MX 2004 For Dummies
  0-7645-4342-3
- FrontPage 2003 For Dummies
  0-7645-3882-9
- HTML 4 For Dummies
  0-7645-1995-6
- Illustrator CS For Dummies
  0-7645-4084-X

- Macromedia Flash MX 2004 For Dummies
  0-7645-4358-X
- Photoshop 7 All-in-One Desk Reference For Dummies
  0-7645-1667-1
- Photoshop CS Timesaving Techniques For Dummies
  0-7645-6782-9
- PHP 5 For Dummies
  0-7645-4166-8
- PowerPoint 2003 For Dummies
  0-7645-3908-6
- QuarkXPress 6 For Dummies
  0-7645-2593-X

NETWORKING, SECURITY, PROGRAMMING & DATABASES

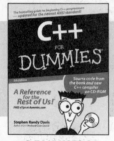

0-7645-6852-3

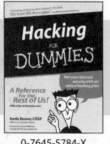

0-7645-5784-X

Also available:
- A+ Certification For Dummies
  0-7645-4187-0
- Access 2003 All-in-One Desk Reference For Dummies
  0-7645-3988-4
- Beginning Programming For Dummies
  0-7645-4997-9
- C For Dummies
  0-7645-7068-4
- Firewalls For Dummies
  0-7645-4048-3
- Home Networking For Dummies
  0-7645-42796

- Network Security For Dummies
  0-7645-1679-5
- Networking For Dummies
  0-7645-1677-9
- TCP/IP For Dummies
  0-7645-1760-0
- VBA For Dummies
  0-7645-3989-2
- Wireless All In-One Desk Reference For Dummies
  0-7645-7496-5
- Wireless Home Networking For Dummies
  0-7645-3910-8

EALTH & SELF-HELP

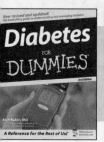

0-7645-6820-5 *†

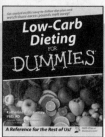

0-7645-2566-2

Also available:
- Alzheimer's For Dummies
  0-7645-3899-3
- Asthma For Dummies
  0-7645-4233-8
- Controlling Cholesterol For Dummies
  0-7645-5440-9
- Depression For Dummies
  0-7645-3900-0
- Dieting For Dummies
  0-7645-4149-8
- Fertility For Dummies
  0-7645-2549-2

- Fibromyalgia For Dummies
  0-7645-5441-7
- Improving Your Memory For Dummies
  0-7645-5435-2
- Pregnancy For Dummies †
  0-7645-4483-7
- Quitting Smoking For Dummies
  0-7645-2629-4
- Relationships For Dummies
  0-7645-5384-4
- Thyroid For Dummies
  0-7645-5385-2

UCATION, HISTORY, REFERENCE & TEST PREPARATION

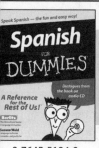

0-7645-5194-9

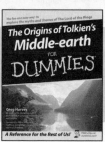

0-7645-4186-2

Also available:
- Algebra For Dummies
  0-7645-5325-9
- British History For Dummies
  0-7645-7021-8
- Calculus For Dummies
  0-7645-2498-4
- English Grammar For Dummies
  0-7645-5322-4
- Forensics For Dummies
  0-7645-5580-4
- The GMAT for Dummies
  0-7645-5251-1
- Inglés Para Dummies
  0-7645-5427-1

- Italian For Dummies
  0-7645-5196-5
- Latin For Dummies
  0-7645-5431-X
- Lewis & Clark For Dummies
  0-7645-2545-X
- Research Papers For Dummies
  0-7645-5426-3
- The SAT I For Dummies
  0-7645-7193-1
- Science Fair Projects For Dummies
  0-7645-5460-3
- U.S. History For Dummies
  0-7645-5249-X

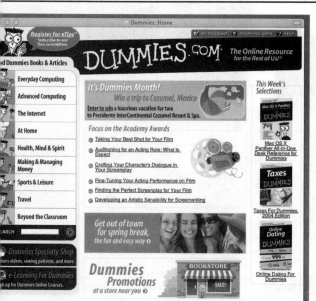

Get smart @ dummies.com®

- **Find a full list of Dummies titles**
- **Look into loads of FREE on-site articles**
- **Sign up for FREE eTips e-mailed to you weekly**
- **See what other products carry the Dummies name**
- **Shop directly from the Dummies bookstore**
- **Enter to win new prizes every month!**

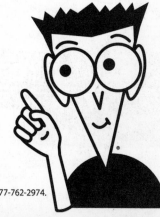

† parate Canadian edition also available
† parate U.K. edition also available

Do More with Dummies
Products for the Rest of Us!

From hobbies to health, discover a wide variety of fun products

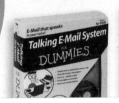
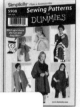
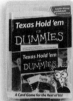
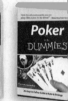

613.7 Tar
Targosz, Cynthia.
Ten minute tone-ups for dummies

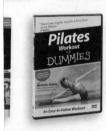
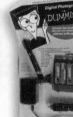
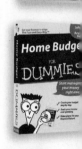

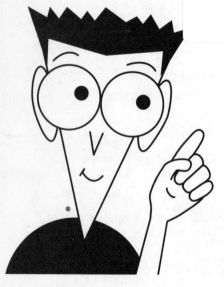

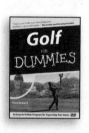
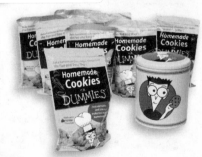

DVDs/Videos • Music CDs • Games
Consumer Electronics • Softwar
Craft Kits • Culinary Kits • and More!

Check out the Dummies Specialty Shop at www.dummies.com for more information!

WILEY